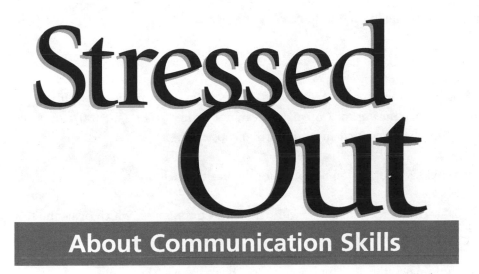

Stressed Out

About Communication Skills

Kathleen Bartholomew, RN, MN

HCPro

Stressed Out About Communication Skills is published by HCPro, Inc.

Copyright © 2007 HCPro, Inc.

ISBN: 978-1-60146-013-4

HCPro, Inc., provides information resources for the healthcare industry.

HCPro, Inc., is not affiliated in any way with The Joint Commission, which owns the JCAHO
and Joint Commission trademarks.

Kathleen Bartholomew, RN, MN, Author

Michael Briddon, Editor

Jamie Gisonde, Executive Editor

Emily Sheahan, Group Publisher

Shane Katz, Cover Designer

Mike Mirabello, Senior Graphic Artist

Michael Roberto, Layout Artist

Chancey Boye, Cartoonist

Leah Tracosas, Copyeditor

Sada Preisch, Proofreader

Darren Kelly, Books Production Supervisor

Susan Darbyshire, Art Director

Claire Cloutier, Production Manager

Jean St. Pierre, Senior Director of Operations

Advice given is general. Readers should consult professional counsel for specific legal, ethical, or
clinical questions.

Arrangements can be made for quantity discounts. For more information, contact:

HCPro, Inc.
75 Sylvan Street, Suite A-101
Danvers, MA 01923
Telephone: 800/650-6787 or 781/639-1872
Fax: 781/639-2982
E-mail: *customerservice@hcpro.com*

Visit the Stressed Out Nurses Web site at: *www.stressedoutnurses.com*

Rev. 09/2011
49725

Dedication

To the wind beneath my wings;
The new nurses and student nurses on our floor
In appreciation and celebration
Of their very presence;
Of their joy and caring competence

Anh Duong
Annette Fly
Skye Heaton
Heidi Jiminez
Jason Malone
Kate Renno
Debra Schrekenghost
Erin Shapleigh
Cheri Yin
Carol McLaughlin

Contents

www.stressedoutnurses.com

How to use this book

What if there was a book that explained complex nursing topics in an easy-to-understand manner and in an accessible format? That's the premise behind the *Stressed Out...series*. Solid references with a bit of a sense of humor and the understanding that a lighthearted approach to learning makes the whole thing more enjoyable.

To help you navigate through the book, you will find the following icons highlighting a particular passage:

Don't panic: Take a deep breath and relax. Get ready for a little reassurance.

Tip: A bit of inside information, a hint, or helpful advice.

Shoes and footprints: Walking in someone else's shoes lets you understand their pain.

Listen up: Powerful examples where effective communication leads to positive change.

Alarm: An instance where poor communication can create dangerous or unhealthy situations.

Happy Nursing! Now you're ready to get started.

About the author

Kathleen Bartholomew, RN, MN

Kathleen Bartholomew, RN, MN, a registered nurse and counselor, uses the power of story from her experience as the manager of a large surgical unit to shed light on the challenges and issues facing nurses today. Her strength is her ability to link the academic world with the practical reality of the hospital. Her objective is to serve as a much-needed voice for nursing today. Bartholomew has been a national speaker for the nursing profession for the past six years. She is also a member of the American Holistic Nurses Association. Recognizing that the culture of an institution is critical to patient safety, she speaks on building community in the workplace and improving nurse-physician relationships. *Speak Your Truth: Proven Strategies for Effective Nurse-Physician Communication* was published by HCPro in 2004 as her Master's thesis. She also wrote the best-selling *Ending Nurse-to-Nurse Hostility: Why Nurses Eat Their Young and Each Other,* also published by HCPro, in 2006. Both her lectures and books reflect her passion and love of nursing.

Acknowledgments

This book wouldn't be possible without Sharon Cox of Cox & Associates of Brentwood, TN. I'd like to give a special thanks to Sharon for her creation of the DESC model, which has helped thousands of nurses to have the conversations necessary to create a healthy work environment.

With recognition and gratitude to Anastasia Hartog, Heidi Jiminez, Diane Mass, Kathleen Tate, Genevieve Bartol, RN, EdD, AHN-C(P), Diana Kraemer, MD, and John Nance, whose supportive feedback I respect and treasure; and appreciation to Martha Griffin, PhD, for her important contributions to new nurses. I would also like to thank Convergent Knowledge Solutions for contributing its information on communication skills and team training.

Introduction

"If not us, then who? If not now, then when?"

The above slogan was used by the organizers of the National Campaign for Improvement of the Volunteer Law in Romania to emphasize the need for immediate action in their society. In America, a similar plea has also been heralded by healthcare advocates. Nowhere is change desperately needed more than in improving communication among healthcare workers.

A recent study by The Joint Commission found that three-fourths of American hospitals cite communication breakdowns as a major cause of devastating sentinel events. In other words, the cause of death was *communication failures*. Communication breakdowns are the cause of 80% of postoperative complications and wrong site, wrong side surgery in The Joint Commission data. For this reason, a National Patient Safety Goal was created stating that hospitals must strive to improve the effectiveness of communication among caregivers. In addition, the American Association of Critical Care Nurses established standards for a healthy work environment which state that "Nurses must be as proficient in communication skills as they are in clinical skills." This is no small task, and for you, it is a clarion call to an added responsibility even at the dawn of your career.

As a nurse, the volume of information that you will receive, process, and act upon in a single shift is daunting. Combine this wealth of data with the fact that you are constantly interrupted and triaging tasks minute by minute, and it's easy to see why communication in the healthcare setting is so challenging—and potentially fatal. That is the purpose and the mission of this book: to give you the tools and methods to effectively communicate.

First, you'll need a crash course in communication basics. After a very brief review of your responsibilities in both sending and receiving information, and listening skills, we'll get straight to play (we can't call it work because you're going to love learning how to connect at a deep and meaningful level with other human beings!)

What are the conversations you avoid? Where do you need more confidence? Talking to a dying patient? Dealing with a coworker who is backstabbing you? Or approaching your manager to talk about a medication error? By the time you are done reading this book, you won't be able to hold yourself back from having these conversations! There is nothing more rewarding than the deep and gratifying feeling of connection that comes from being able to convey your own thoughts and feelings *and* understand the thoughts and feelings of others. Every time this happens, you weave an invisible thread, until the fabric of your life becomes a tapestry of deep, meaningful, rich, and colorful relationships.

Part One

As nurses, we all have a desire to help people. And to help them, we must be able to communicate with them. This section will lay out some common communication errors and give you essential tips for dealing with difficult patients. The bedside will never be the same again.

Chapter 1

Communication 101

> "The greatest enemy of effective communication is the illusion of it."
>
> —Daryl R. Smith, *Controlling Pilot Error*

Communication is the process of exchanging information. Information is conveyed as words, tone of voice, and body language. But studies have shown that words account for only 7% of the information communicated! Vocal tone accounts for 55% and body language accounts for 38%. To be effective communicators, you need to be aware of your words, tone of voice, and body language at all times.

Sender responsibilities

Both the sender and the receiver have specific responsibilities if communication is to be effective. The sender must ensure that he or she is clear, concise, and to the point, and must also pay attention to background noise. Do not hesitate to move out of the nurse's station or congested areas if necessary. It is also your responsibility to notice if the receiver is receptive to the information you are conveying.

The sender should:

- State one idea at a time
- State ideas simply and clearly
- Monitor his or her tone of voice and tempo
- Explain when appropriate
- Repeat if necessary (if he or she sees ANY doubt!)
- Encourage feedback—ask if the receiver is getting the message
- Read between the lines: Does your choice of words, tone, and body language all convey the same meaning?

Receiver responsibilities

The receiver also has a set of communication responsibilities. Most people will not really listen or pay attention to your point of view until they become convinced you have heard—and appreciate—theirs (Nichols). Be aware of your overload point and stop the transmission if necessary. You could ask the sender to slow down, or stop and say that you want to write the information down. If the information is not urgent, put the sender on hold (just like a telephone.) Listen carefully and provide feedback—acknowledge whether you understand the message, or you don't. If you don't "get it," ask the sender to say it a different way or to say it again. Then, repeat what you think you heard.

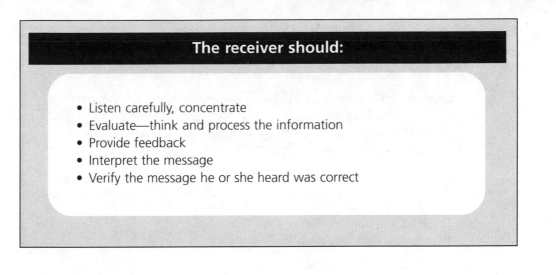

The receiver should:

- Listen carefully, concentrate
- Evaluate—think and process the information
- Provide feedback
- Interpret the message
- Verify the message he or she heard was correct

Open your ears

"A wise old owl sat on an oak;
The more he saw the less he spoke;
The less he spoke the more he heard;
Why aren't we like that wise old bird?"

—Author unknown

We grow up with the mistaken belief that listening is a "no-brainer," when, in fact, listening is a learned skill you can practice and get better at with time. On average, a physician will interrupt a patient describing his or her symptoms within 18 seconds of meeting that patient. *In that short time,* many doctors decide on the likely diagnosis and best treatment (Groopman). We talk at 125–250 words per minute, but can listen at 450–900 words per minute! Studies show that immediately after listening to someone, we recall only 50% of what was said. Here are some techniques to practice that will improve your listening skills:

- Focus on what's being said *and not* your response.

- Body language: Assess your body positioning for a listening stance. There's a big difference between a nod and crossing your arms!

- Reflective feedback: Ask questions, or make brief statements that show you understand the message. Don't hesitate to ask for a repeat if necessary. If the subject matter is complex, repeat back to the sender what you think you heard.

- Eye contact is critical. It tells the sender you are following the message.

- Silence can be very effective as well, and tells the sender you are processing the information or that you want more information. People will often volunteer more details when given the opportunity.

- Pull out action items, especially immediate or critical tasks. Repeat them out loud at the end of the conversation. For example: *"You want me to go to pharmacy and pick up the Fentanyl PCA and bring it to the nurse who is taking care of the patient in room 966? Correct?"*

Become aware of what you communicate

> *"By three methods we may learn wisdom:*
> *First, by reflection, which is noblest;*
> *Second, by imitation, which is easiest;*
> *And third, by experience, which is the most bitter."*
>
> —Confucius

Here's the interesting part: If words comprise only 7% of communication, then tone of voice and body language make up the other 93%! The nonverbal messages that the pitch of your voice and your body posturing send out are as loud as a foghorn. So what's the problem? The sender is focused on the words and is completely unaware that his or her body is relaying the "real message." (You think you are on a private line, when in fact, the speakerphone has been on all the time.) **Nonverbal communication broadcasts our true feelings to the world.** Your body is shouting what your conscious mind thinks it's hiding!

Confusion rules the conversation as people respond to the nonverbal message you didn't know you were sending.

The essence of communication, therefore, becomes self-awareness. There is a direct relationship between the degree to which we can effectively communicate with others, and the degree to which we know ourselves. The more we become aware of our own feelings, thoughts, and motivations, the more easily we will be able to perceive the thoughts, feelings, and motivations of others. The more real-life experiences we are exposed to, the more opportunities we have to learn and grow. It's not always about what you say. It's about who you are. There is just no faking 93% of the message.

Experience doesn't always have to be firsthand and bitter. You can learn from the experiences of others. The narratives and examples in this book were selected after surveying student and new nurses and asking them, "What are the hardest conversations for you to have with your patients, peers, physicians, and your manager?" Curious?

Critical situations that demand a conversation

A study from VitalSmarts describes the conversations that healthcare professionals struggle with that contribute to patient harm and unacceptable error rates:

Broken rules—shortcuts, not following procedures, neglecting double-checks

Mistakes—poor clinical judgment, inadequate assessment, failure to triage correctly

Lack of support—complaining, refusing to help or share information, criticism

Incompetence—lack of knowledge and skills, poor standard of care

Poor teamwork—cliques, unhealthy competition, upstaging, not valuing team members, blame

Disrespect—condescending language, rudeness, dismissive remarks, slamming education or experience of others

Micromanagement—bullying, threat or force due to misuse of authority

Adapted from "Silence Kills: The Seven Crucial Conversations® for Healthcare"

Chapter 2

The art of compassionate nursing

> "The most basic and powerful way to connect to another person is to listen. Just listen. Perhaps the most important thing we ever give each other is our attention. . . . A loving silence often has far more power to heal and to connect than the most well-intentioned words."
>
> —Rachel Naomi Remen

One of your nursing school instructors' primary focuses was to teach you the information required to pass the NCLEX. This curriculum represents the science of nursing and is the foundation of knowledge for our profession. The rationale gleaned from this science guides all critical thinking and decision-making.

But there is much more. No doubt you have heard senior nurses say their "real" education began the minute they graduated. As a new nurse, you too will experience all of the information and theory from nursing school coming alive—from a two-dimensional black-and-white print to a three-dimensional hologram. For example, instead of reading about types of psychiatric illnesses, someone in your care is severely depressed. Now "the depressed patient" has a name—and that, in itself, makes all the difference in the world.

No book could ever give you all of the appropriate words to handle the myriad situations you will encounter. Each individual's life experience is profoundly unique and does not lend itself to convenient categories. Life itself becomes your next teacher. If you know a few key points, your interactions with your patients will teach you the "art" of nursing. Inherent in this art is the ability to connect with all human beings. What are some of these stories? And how can you prepare yourself to communicate effectively *no matter what* the situation?

 ## Patients: In their shoes

> *"Never judge another until you have walked three miles in their moccasins."*
>
> —Indian proverb

As it turns out, there is simply no place more dangerous to be than a hospital. Since 1999, the general public has known that hospital errors kill more people every year than cancer, AIDS, or motor vehicle accidents. Hospital mistakes account for 44,000–98,000 deaths every year. To put it in perspective, if a Boeing 747 filled with passengers crashed every Monday, Wednesday, and Friday for an entire year, that would only account for the *lowest* estimated figure of 44,000 deaths.

In January 2007, *USA Today* ran an article that advised patients to look out for their own well-being in the hospital. One of the suggestions in the article was that patients ask caregivers to wash their hands—good advice, considering the fact that 150 patients die every single day of nosocomial infections (those acquired during the hospital stay). The Centers for Disease Control and Prevention estimates the annual number of infections at about 90,000. To make matters worse, another recent study found that only 48% of physicians comply with handwashing regulations. But when a patient is sick and knocked out on pain medications, it can be difficult to remember to tell caregivers to wash their hands. Within a week, a *USA Today* editorial read, "Why should patients be the vigilantes of their own care when they are the ones who need watching over?" Good question.

Still, patients continue to place their trust in us, though any nurse can tell you patients' fear and anxiety levels have increased dramatically. They are confused and forgetful due to medications or illness and feel terribly apprehensive. In this fog, they struggle to understand why they are taking new medications or having procedures done. Many have read newspaper stories about fatal hospital mistakes and know that every patient experiences a medication error *at a minimum* of once a shift. Patients are anxious.

Patients also feel vulnerable. For example, many elderly female patients are embarrassed to have a male caregiver help them in the bathroom or with bathing but hesitate to say anything unless prompted. They hide their embarrassment and are slow to complain, fearing retaliation.

Hospital administrators struggle to meet financial targets; physicians try to manage falling reimbursements; and nurses struggle to meet the patient's physical, emotional, and psychological needs. But it's the patient who feels the brunt of a system when it does not work.

Hospitalized patients feel a profound sense of helplessness. They often cannot move, eat, or void without assistance, and they depend on their caregivers for the most basic of all needs. Their apprehension level increases tremendously when a call light is not answered or they can't find their call light. They see their bed as a prison to which the nurse holds the key. Patients feel helpless, scared, anxious, and vulnerable. Who wouldn't?

The old man's fight

The old man was fighting death as if it were a bull. He tossed and turned in his bed day and night, trying to dodge the big beast. The family was exhausted (as they had been at his bedside for days) and extremely embarrassed because this well-educated, genteel man was cursing profusely. "We have never heard him cuss even once in his entire life," said his wife, mortified. When the doctor rounded on day three, he was surprised to find his patient still alive. After observing the patient, he ordered a sedative.

Still, the old man continued to fight with his bed covers and ramble incoherently. On the fourth day, he found himself in the care of a new nurse who decided that while she was giving him his bath she would listen to every single muttered word—no matter how strange. A good 20 minutes later, a smile of contentment came over her face. She had put the incoherent babbling words together as if they were a jigsaw puzzle, grabbing pieces here and there to finally solve the mystery.

This was what she could make out: When the old man was only 19 and a sailor, he had gone to a brothel. Now, he was terrified that he was going "straight to hell." There was no way out. He had spent his whole life doing good, trying to make up for his mistake.

The nurse stroked the patient's forehead and struggled to meet his wild gaze. Firmly, she said, "Listen to me. I know God is loving—you are not going to hell!" He stopped squirming, so she repeated the words again.

"No, no," the old man said, with more pity than hope.

"Yes, yes," the nurse replied. "I know about the brothel. You are not going to hell. You are a good man."

The old man's breathing became shallower. Finally, he stopped rambling and squirming. "Good man," he repeated softly. "Good man."

The family remarked to the nurse how calm their father seemed after the bath. Within the hour, he passed.

It is an honor to be with another human being when he or she is the most vulnerable. Consider it a privilege to stand witness to the most intimate moments of life. Nurses work at the portal of the planet, assisting new beings as they enter and leave our world; facilitating healing; and providing comfort, caring, and support to people of all cultures, all religions, and all manner of dispositions.

Making the connection

As a nurse graduate (or someone headed in that direction), you already possess a basic knowledge of communication skills. Most of the time, patients seem rational enough. You can relate to your patients using many of the tools and information you learned in school: assessing for readiness to learn, asking for verbalization, and validating understanding. Most of the time, you can connect with your patient and work together to accomplish the goals set forth in the plan of care.

But patients are not always rational. Their feelings often override any conscious thought when they find themselves in a vulnerable situation, and they act out by being nonconforming, rebellious, extremely needy, etc. Everyday encounters can become extremely frustrating, and your goals for the day can seem to move further out of reach with each hour. In these situations, knowing what to do can be an enormous challenge because the patient does not respond to reason.

> *"The heart has its reason that reason knows not."*
>
> —Blaise Pascal

However, realize that patients almost always respond to caring. No matter what their experience, gender, culture, or situation, all humans know the language of the heart. It is this ability to connect heart-to-heart that will give you the supreme confidence to know that you can handle any situation, no matter how formidable. This is the art of nursing: connecting with caring and compassion.

Communication is the tool by which we connect. To use this tool, listening, presence, and a nonjudgmental attitude are required. Words, believe it or not, are optional.

Ready, set, listen

As Rachel Naomi Remen says, "the most powerful way to connect to another person is to listen." Sometimes we *think* we are listening because we hear the words. But you can hear words and miss their message. Listening is the active process of interpreting, evaluating, and responding to what was said. Patients will know whether you listened or not the minute they hear your response.

Taking the time to listen can be a tremendous challenge when you are faced with a list of tasks to complete by the end of your shift. Time is a very real constraint, and new nurses often say what they miss the most are the conversations they used to have as a student nurse with their patients. Over time, tasks will become more repetitive, and you will eventually find that you once again have the time to be an attentive listener and engage your patients' hearts and souls.

Chapter 3

Aim for the heart

In my role as nurse manager, I have visited over a thousand patient rooms asking questions about patient care: Did your care meet your expectations? Is there something we could have done to make your stay better? It is the thousand answers to these questions that have taught me the most about nurse-patient communication.

Quite simply put, patients either like their nurses or they don't. Lukewarm responses are rare. After listening to countless stories, it all comes down to only one thing: Patients respond to the nurse who shows them that he or she cares.

 Alarm: Mary had been on our unit for almost a year. She did well clinically and was always on top of her patients' plan of care, consistently using critical thinking to advocate for her patients' needs. Yet, not once in the entire year did the manager ever receive a patient compliment about her nursing. Curious, the manager visited a few of Mary's patients prior to her performance evaluation. She discovered that Mary was as proficient as an android. According to patients, she went through the steps of nursing like a robot who memorized a dance routine. The patients' perception was that "Mary just doesn't care," or, as one patient put it, "I didn't know that you could be a nurse and not care."

When the manager shared the patients' feedback, Mary was perplexed. She struggled to understand what was missing, and when she could not find the caring inside, signed up for counseling. Mary couldn't give what she didn't have.

 Tip: Often, even though most nurses *do care* very much, the patients' perception is *that their nurses do not care*. This usually happens when patients perceive that a nurse is in a hurry and when there is little eye contact, touching, or small talk. Forcing yourself to slow down for just five minutes to connect with your patient will have a noticeable effect on the entire shift.

To love the world, you must first love yourself

> *"Healing happens more easily through us when we allow it to happen in us."*
>
> —Frances Vaughan

All the book knowledge in the world could not give Mary the thing she needed most—self-love. For communication to be therapeutic, **you *must* have a deep sense of compassion and love for yourself**. "The more nurses become healed and whole themselves, the more they have to offer their patients. As they grow and develop in self-love and compassion, their well of compassion and mercy for others expands" (Quinn). It is this well of empathy that is most healing to patients. Knowing that someone is willing to be with them in their time of need, anger, fear, or loss can make all the difference.

The quality of your relationship with your patient is directly related to the relationship you have with yourself. For example, if you have ever lost a child, that can resonate profoundly with another mother who has also lost a child—your patient feels this instinctively. If you find yourself criticizing and judging a patient, there is a good chance you don't forgive yourself for a similar mistake. Compassion and criticism can't exist in the same space.

Tip: If you find yourself being critical, stop and rewind. Is there an association between this patient's situation and a past event in your life? Look at this moment as an opportunity for your growth and healing.

Tip: Keep "self-care" at the top of your priority list. Listen to what you need—body, mind, and soul. Your most important patient is you. Take breaks, stay hydrated, and breathe deep. The intensity of the job will ebb and flow—to keep from "drowning" you've got to ride the waves.

Presence is a present

> *"Come into the conversation with empty hands. Bring nothing but yourself."*
>
> —Susan Scott

The last thing you need in communicating with patients is words. It's like having a cell phone that's not connected to any service: If you don't have a signal, it really doesn't matter what you say. Every time you walk into a patient's room, your very presence sends off a vibration. Be aware of the nonverbal signals you are sending; if you are not, the patient will react, but you won't have any idea what he or she is reacting to! You are transparent. Even though you might not say the words out loud, the vibration comes through loud and clear . . .

Alarm: "I don't have time to chat—it's already 10 a.m., and I'm not finished the med pass . . ."
"Great, a homeless person. The bath will take an hour . . . "
"I need to hurry because 967 needs pain meds . . ."

By its nature, nursing involves a tremendous amount of multitasking. You assess the color and quantity of urine in the Foley catheter while you are hanging the IV, all while you're talking to the patient and trying to listen for the physician you just paged. Being present with a patient these days is challenging for *even the most experienced of nurses*. Here are some tips for staying present when you walk into a patient's room:

- Try to jot down as much as you possibly can in your notes. Don't try to keep a "to-do" list in your head (*especially* the little things, such as replacing a box of tissues). Trying to remember *everything* will take your attention away from *everyone*.

- Stop at the doorway and take two or three long, deep breaths.

- Be keenly aware. The most important communication happens within the first minute of walking into the room—*whether anyone speaks or not*.

- *Before* you speak, look patients directly in the eye and touch them lightly on the hand or leg—or touch the bed covers (depending on your comfort level and the patient's receptiveness).

- Focus in on the particular patient—*not* "room 542," *not* "the pneumonia patient."

- Communication is primarily nonverbal. What does the patient's body position tell you? What would you feel like if you were in that position?

- Pay attention to the surroundings: Is the room messy or neat? Are there any flowers or cards? What does the environment say? What is it like to be in this room?

Listen up: The patient had terminal cancer. When I entered the room she was sitting in a chair, staring out the window. But as soon as she saw me, she closed her eyes, shutting me out of her world.

It took several minutes to change the bed and clean up the room. During this time, I said nothing, but thought about how I would feel if I was in her position. Suddenly she stood up, and I helped her back into the bed, fixing her pillow and tucking the bed covers around her chin without a word. Then I said a prayer and tried to grasp the sorrow in her eyes.

It was just as I turned to leave that she finally spoke. Suddenly, she reached out and grabbed my hand, catching me off guard.

"Don't think for a minute that I am unaware of all you have done for me. Thank you."

"You're welcome," I said, half-wondering myself what it was that I supposedly did.

This nurse did a lot. She picked up right away on the fact that the patient was not open to small talk (she shut her eyes). She was also comfortable with the silence and emotionally present to the patient the entire time she was in the room. This nurse was willing simply to be with the patient in her feelings of loss and grief as she tried to take in the reality of her illness—and the patient felt and appreciated the company.

> *"I want to know if you can sit with pain, mine or your own, without moving to hide it, or fade it, or fix it."*
>
> —Oriah Mountain Dreamer

You cannot define or interpret an experience for someone else. You can't always make things better. What you can do, however, is to simply stay—and sometimes that is the hardest part. That means not trying to change, fix, improve, or heal, but just *being* with your patient as this scene in the story of his or her life unfolds so the patient doesn't have to be alone.

We are, by nature, communal beings. We need each other. Patients can be surrounded by visitors and caregivers and still feel an acute loneliness because no one is willing or brave enough to stay with them as they travel through a fog of emotions. The feelings patients experience are intense and unfamiliar. But when someone *is willing* to stay with them, to stand witness to their unique experience, it is *more than* "enough"—presence is the ultimate service.

Keep an open mind

 Alarm: "My first quarter, 5th time in clinical, I had to care for a patient who was just released from jail. It was difficult to get certain thoughts out of my head . . . 'What did he do?'"

Alarm: "Conversations about abuse and STDs are just really hard for me."

Patients will pick up on your fears or prejudices faster than you are even aware of them. Your body does not lie. Your patients are a mirror. Their intuition immediately interprets your subtly raised eyebrow or the few extra inches you create between you and them. No less compassion and understanding is required of a nurse than if he or she were a rabbi or minister.

So what can you do?

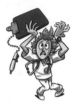

Don't panic: As soon as you read a diagnosis, or hear something about a patient that produces an "ugh" or "yuck" within, take some extra time before you go into the room.

- **Search:** Scan your past like a recorder on rewind for any personal history. Just being aware of a past experience will help tremendously.

- **Personalize:** *Always* call the patient by his or her name, and ask the patient what he or she would like to be called.

- **Imagine:** Put yourself in the patient's place. What must it feel like to be this patient under these circumstances?

- **Be curious:** What is this patient's unique story? Sometimes you may have to do some searching. What is something you both have in common?

- **Remember:** Your value system is just that—*yours*.

Listen up: The 25-year-old drug addict had been living on the street for eight years. Because she had methicillin-resistant Staphylococcus aureus (MRSA), she was placed on isolation, which immediately decreased staff interaction time. Her hand had been cut and was badly infected. The doctor had to open and drain the wound in the ER. Now nursing hung IV antibiotics and performed wet-to-dry dressings twice a day.

Every nurse on the floor would tell you that they treated her "just like every other patient." Yet, they made comments when the skinny girl ordered seven trays of food a day. It was the look on their faces that betrayed them as much as their lack of anything nice to say.

On the seventh hospital day, a new nurse entered the room. The patient was brusque and bossy and began ordering the nurse around. So the nurse stopped what she was doing right away and said, "I can tell you really know what's going on, so why don't I just set everything up and then you can tell me what to do step-by-step." This pleased the patient, whose name was Sarah—and also pleased the experienced nurse who could see Sarah soften ever so slightly after given total control over the procedure.

During the procedure, the nurse started asking Sarah questions: "How long have you been on the street? What do you do? Do you ever want to go home?" Sarah swelled with pride. She told the nurse it was her job to send runaways back to their parents. This was her mission, her "purpose in life," and it was "very, very important." She explained that the cut hand was a result of trying to protect a young teenager from being sold a dirty needle.

The nurse, of course, told Sarah's story to everyone—and the nurses no longer "treated her just like any other patient."

Still uncomfortable? Imagine that this patient is a family member—your sister or father, etc. It stretches the heart open a little farther and helps you empathize. When you have time, write a small paragraph about what it must feel like to be this particular patient.

Remember, judgmental, derogatory comments about a patient go against the basic tenet of nursing practice: respect for all individuals despite their situation or diagnosis. Have you ever noticed how one derogatory comment acts like an open invitation for other comments? Bad comments are contagious.

 Tip: Don't tolerate derogatory comments about a patient from anyone.

Caring . . .

. . . is a nurturing way of relating to a valued other toward whom one feels a personal sense of commitment and responsibility.

Caring process	definition	expressions
MAINTAINING BELIEF	sustaining faith in the other's capacity to get through an event or transition and face a future with meaning	believing in/holding in esteem maintaining a hope-filled attitude offering realistic optimism "going the distance" helping find meaning
KNOWING	striving to understand an event as it has meaning in the life of another	avoiding assumptions centering on the one cared-for assessing thoroughly seeking cues engaging the self of both
BEING WITH	being emotionally present to the other	being there conveying availability enduring with sharing feelings not burdening
DOING FOR	doing for the other as he or she would do for the self if it were at all possible	comforting anticipating performing competently/skillfully protecting preserving dignity
ENABLING	facilitating the other's passage through life transitions and unfamiliar events	informing/explaining supporting/allowing focusing generating alternatives/thinking it through validating/giving feedback

Source: Adapted from Kristen M. Swanson, RN, PhD, FAAN. Used with permission.

Chapter 4

Can you hear me now? Common communication errors

Nurses go into the profession because they want to help people. They have an intense desire to make things better. They want the pain to go away, the patient to sleep comfortably, and the illness to be cured. Then they feel good about themselves, as well.

So it's challenging then when things don't go as planned. Sometimes patients simply won't comply with the regimen that you know will heal them. This situation often leaves both the nurse and the patient frustrated. At the source of our frustration are some basic assumptions that we seldom verbalize. Many nurses come into the profession believing:

- Everyone wants to get better.

- Health is good. Death/disease are bad.

- I did listen. I can repeat every word.

- There must be *something* I can do.

- It's my job to fix the situation and make it better.

- There is an appropriate response for every situation.

These assumptions will set us up for failure if we don't check them out and acknowledge their influence on our practice. They are the source of some of the most common nurse-patient communication errors:

1. Nurses respond to what was said instead of to the underlying feeling

2. Nurses feel rejected—they take patient comments personally and feel like they have failed when the patient is difficult

3. Nurses feel a profound sense of helplessness when they can't fix the problem or find a solution

Healing doesn't always mean health. Some patients experience a profound healing even though the clinical outcome is chronic disease or even death. For example, their illness might have helped them to face their worst fears or to heal damage to a long-standing relationship.

Dying doesn't always mean death. Some patients may recover physically but not emotionally, psychologically, or spiritually. They cannot (or will not) recover from a great loss or make sense of a devastating illness. They are filled with a resentment and rage, which slowly drains the life force from them.

Tip: Don't make assumptions. Things are not always as they seem.

Nurse huddle . . . Here are some secrets

Sometimes, patients put up a strong front for family members because they don't want to worry them. Then, as soon as the family leaves, fears and insecurities set in like a fog and patients are engulfed in a typhoon of emotions. Here are some examples:

• Patients who know that their families are having trouble coping with their impending death will not die until the family has had time to adjust or a relative has finally arrived.

• Some patients' pain will get better the second a family member leaves the room, and some patients' pain will get much worse.

• Patients who have been fiercely independent their whole lives struggle with their sudden dependence and often refuse to call for help.

• Other patients ring the call light repeatedly because they can't reach a tissue box only four inches from their hand.

Respond to the feeling tone

Alarm: As soon as the day nurse walked into the room, her patient, who was a recent quadriplegic, started complaining. Irritated, the man said, "I asked for a glass of water at 2 a.m. and that night nurse made me wait until almost 6 a.m.!"

How do you respond?

- **DON'T** fall into the trap of justifying or protecting the night nurse:

  "Oh, I am sure she must have had an emergency and forgot."

- **DON'T** agree with the patient:

  "She sure did make you wait a long time. I'm sorry."

- **DO** respond to the feeling tone (which is helplessness):

  "It must feel awful to be dependent on someone else for something as simple as a drink of water." The key is to respond to the feeling. Then, the floodgates will open . . .

Listen up: The 32-year-old female patient learned from her doctor that morning that the brain tumor was a glioma—"like Jell-O in the brain." He had said, "We just can't get it out." The doctor proposed a plan: The patient would stay in the hospital for 48 hours and receive osmolytes to shrink her brain. Then, she would go home with hospice care.

Less than three hours later, the patient rang the call light and shouted angrily, "No one is doing anything about my brain tumor!" The nurse promised to come to her room in five minutes, as soon as she had given the pain meds in her hand to another patient.

But while she was still down the hall, the patient started yelling again—and this time, she didn't bother to use the call light. She just screamed at the top of her lungs, and the entire floor could hear her.

Quickly, the nurse rushed into the room just as the patient was taking a gulp of air to yell again. As soon as she saw the patient she abruptly said, "Do you like chocolate-covered strawberries?"

The patient paused for a moment and then answered very matter-of-factly, "Why, yes. Yes I do."

"Great," said the nurse. "Please order a bowl of strawberries and three Hershey bars and call me when they get here. I'll melt the chocolate in the microwave, and you can hand-dip the berries." The patient dialed nutrition and placed the order.

The *words* were: "No one is doing anything about my brain tumor!"
The *feeling* was: "I am desperate because I've lost all control . . . HELPLESS!"

The nurse gave her what no medication ever could—some semblance of control in her life when she felt like she was free-falling from 30,000 feet without a parachute. After having the chocolate-covered strawberries, the patient and the nurse worked together to make a plan of care for discharge. The patient identified eight things she wanted to do before she died and wrote them herself on a clipboard the nurse provided. She returned to the hospital in a coma three months later. The family found the nurse because they wanted to tell her that the patient had "done everything on the list."

Take a look from a different perspective

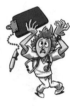

Don't panic: "What do you do when your patient seems obsessively focused on himself or herself?"

Reframe the situation. Help patients to see their situation from a different perspective. In the movie *Moonstruck*, Cher (who plays the heroine) meets her future brother-in-law and discovers that he is mired in self-pity because of an accident that cost him his arm and his fiancée. She listens attentively as he vents his fury and tells his story.

Then Cher takes the same events and reworks the story. She gives her brother-in-law a present he will use every minute for the rest of his life: a new way to see the situation. She tells him that he is a "wolf"—a wolf who found himself in a trap (engaged to the wrong woman). The accident in which he lost his hand was not really an accident, but rather a desperate bid for freedom. In fact, he bit off his hand to save himself from a marriage that would have been a terrible mistake. Cher tells him:

"You are a wolf. You were caught in a trap and headed for marriage—and to think that you bit off your own hand to free yourself!"

The brother-in-law's body responds first to the words. Immediately, his back stiffens as he straightens up, feeling great pride, taking on the idea that there must've been a part of him that wanted desperately to get out of this marriage. He likes this new story.

Every patient wants to make sense of his or her own illness. Patients want desperately to understand the answer to the question, "Why me?" Hospital-izations and illnesses are not planned life events. Patients suddenly find themselves waking up one morning to horrendous crises, feeling extremely vulnerable and helpless. For example, many fear the effect of their absence on their career or worry about losing their jobs. Mothers worry about how to care for their children. Because nurses see sick people every day, we sometimes forget just how stressful illness can be.

 Tip: When humans perform repetitive acts day after day, once-special tasks soon become routine. What was once scary to a new grad or student can quickly become routine—but it is *always* unfamiliar to the patient.

A reframing case study

When Cassie, the nurse, entered the room, the 42-year-old woman was writhing in pain, holding her stomach and moaning. Cassie was alerted to the patient by the blinking call light. As she entered the room she said, "Can I help you?"

The patient angrily lashed out at Cassie. "God help me. Don't tell me you're my nurse—because you don't know a damn thing. Read the chart, girl. I have three ulcers! How come I get all the stupid nurses?" And then she went back to her moaning and writhing.

Cassie ignored the patient's criticism and harsh words and instead acted with genuine curiosity. She could tell by her patient's exaggerated movements that she was very focused on her situation. Perhaps she could do something to break the spell?

Cassie calmly went over to the whiteboard and picked up the magic marker while erasing the board. With an even tone she said, "What are their names?"

The patient was indignant. "What are you talking about? I have no idea what you are talking about."

"Oh, just give it a try," cajoled Cassie while drawing large, medium, and small circles on the whiteboard.

The patient stopped moving and looked for just a second at the circles Cassie had drawn. Then, still staring out the window, the patient said adamantly, "The largest one is my ex-husband—Bob." Cassie filled in the name "Bob" in the largest circle and waited.

Immediately, the patient's whole body language shifted. Instead of being angry and helpless, the patient was now curious too about the connection between the stress in her life and her ulcers.

A few minutes later the patient added, "And the smallest one is my bills—the finances are a mess." No longer was the patient writhing in bed. Now, she had something to think about, something she just might be able to control—her stress.

Chapter 5

Difficult patients: Between a rock and a hard place

> *"The increase in aggressive behaviors within healthcare delivery systems mirrors the violence in our society. . . . Of all healthcare providers, nurses face the greatest risk of encountering aggressive patients' acts."*
>
> —Leslie Nield-Anderson, APRN, PhD

Depressed . . . rebellious . . . psychotic . . . confused . . . isolated . . . angry . . . demeaning . . . patients.

It's an incredible and extremely rewarding challenge to deal with every color on the humanity spectrum—*without a psychiatrist prescription pad!* Keep in mind that people are trying the best they can to deal with their particular situations. Here are some basic tips for the most challenging patients:

- Establish a relationship—realize that this bond is your most therapeutic tool.

- Encourage sharing of feelings. Suggest coping strategies, if the patient is receptive.

- Name the dragon! That is, validate the emotion. Say, "You seem angry, depressed, etc."

- Always respond to the feeling tone and not the words.

- Ask the patient what he or she needs. Don't assume.

- Always give the patient as much control as possible.

 Alarm: Some of the most common ways patients exert control are by being demanding, rebellious, or needy.

Coping with anger!

Every time I walk into a room to de-escalate a patient, I can't help but wonder how we missed the clues: What were the early signs of agitation that were missed? At what point could we have intervened sooner to calm this person and assuage his or her fears? Patients typically progress in their anger until they are "on fire" with emotion—from being annoyed and irritated, on to being angry, and then finally to being in a full-blown rage. What fuels this emotional fire? The key is to pay attention to the early clues. It's a lot easier to blow out a match than to douse a bonfire. Look for agitation, sleeplessness, radical mood swings, sources of tension, and general irritability. Bring these behaviors to the patient's attention and focus on the event that triggered the feeling. Assess the medication regimen and ask for a psychological consult if the event is sudden and you can't identify a trigger.

 Tip: The goal of this communication is to help the patient pinpoint the emotional trigger.

Just below the surface of every raging patient is pain, fear, or loss. Anger is often a secondary emotion people use when they can't deal with pain, when they feel trapped, or during the normal process of grief.

Here are some very important dos and don'ts you should know when dealing with aggressive patients (Anderson and Clarke):

DO!
- Speak in a lower tone of voice than the patient.

- Move to a private place where others can see you. If you are in the patient's room, stand where you are visible from the doorway. Or, go to the corner of a large room.

- Alert the charge nurse to the situation.

- Assume the same position as the patient—for example, sit if they are sitting.

- Call security for backup. Just knowing they are available helps.

- Listen. Use the patient's own words in conversation.

- Paraphrase what the patient is angry about.

- Ask open-ended questions.

- Direct the conversation to the primary emotion and empathize.

- Validate the emotion. Name it: "You sound furious."

- Move toward a behavioral contract (a document stating which behaviors are acceptable), if necessary, after the incident cools down.

- Ask for cooperation and state the common goal.

- Ask for a psych consult if you can't determine the trigger or if you are uncertain.

- Document the event.

DON'T!

- Don't sound judgmental, blame, make excuses, or argue.

- *Never* touch an angry patient—give him or her space.

- Don't make any sudden moves.

- Don't show up in force—keep your backup discreet.

- Don't cross your arms or point at the patient. Keep your hands visible and be aware of your body language.

- *Never* let the patient get between you and the door.

Tip: Nothing aggravates a patient more than having to tell every single nurse the same thing over and over again. Their interpretation is that "no one cares enough to remember." *Write down* patients' personal requests or accommodations on the Kardex or in the nurses' notes (e.g., "Mr. Smith feels claustrophobic—keep windows and doors open," etc.) The little things *do* count.

Tip: Difficult patients can exhaust even the most experienced nurses. If you feel overwhelmed, drained, or anxious just anticipating your day, then it's *not* your day to have the difficult patient again. Don't hesitate to ask the charge nurse to relieve you of that patient—and don't forget to pass along everything you've learned.

Tip: At the same time, realize it's easier when the patient and caregiver have known each other. Caregiver continuity is the goal *if you have the energy.* Familiarity breeds security.

Rebellious, resistant, and refusing to cooperate

Alarm: In the discharge instructions, the cancer patient was told she was not allowed to eat spinach. But as soon as she was discharged, she went straight to the store, bought a large bunch of spinach, went home, and ate it for dinner.

Sometimes, when the cards are stacked against you, all you want to do is knock them down—just because you can. Being noncompliant or refusing to cooperate is a common way for patients to rebel—they feel like they've finally found something they can control. When circumstances are out of your control, such as during an illness, it's scary. Address the feelings (insecurity, helplessness, etc.) and always try to give the patient as much control as possible. Even the little things like decisions on when to take a bath or a pill can make a big difference.

Patients with oppositional behavior act like children who are testing their limits. Just as children feel more secure when the parent takes control, patients who are rebellious or defiant need security, and caregivers give patients that security by setting limits (Renno).

Tip: Set boundaries. Clearly state what behaviors are unacceptable.

Tip: Make a compromise. Focus the conversation on a goal the patient wants (washing his or her hair)—then add a goal you would like to accomplish (giving a suppository). Ask the patient which goal he or she wants to accomplish first and offer options (e.g., ask whether you and the patient should tackle the goals now or after lunch). Every time you give patients an option, you are giving them control.

Tip: Start with the things you know the patient will do. Always give instructions in threes; for example, "Take a deep breath; wiggle your toes; give me your arm," etc. By giving short, simple instructions, you set up an unconscious pattern of cooperation (commonly used in hypnosis).

Here are some more hot tips from the experts:

- Decide how important this particular compliance situation is (there's a big difference between refusing a stool softener and refusing an antibiotic). If it's not a big deal, then respect their right to refuse.

- Sometimes it helps for patients to see the care pathway and the goals for a particular day. Then, they can see how the activity fits into the total plan.

- It really, really helps for the patient to understand the rationale.

- I give a pep talk—"Come on, let's give it a try" or "You'll feel so much better."

- I use a lot of humor. For example, when the patient refuses their foot pumps I say, "Hum, tough choice, foot pumps or blood clot?"

Dealing with unrealistic expectations

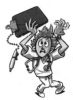

Don't panic: "How do you handle extremely needy patients?"

Needy patients are convinced there is no one on the unit but them—or at least no one that needs you as much as they do. They are the center of their own universe, and sometimes it feels as if their goal is only to see how fast you can spin.

The key to dealing with demanding patients is to realize their behavior stems from a fear of abandonment. Senior nurses have learned some important tips (Hagedorn):

- Meet the patient head on. On the very first visit, spend *extra time* with needy patients so they feel more secure. The more time you spend up-front, the better the entire shift will be.

- Ask questions that show you want to know who the patient is as a person because you care. Just being "known" fosters security.

- Answer lights promptly. It decreases anxiety and reassures the patient you will be there when he or she needs you.

- Do everything you can think of while you are in the room and always ask: "Is there anything else I can do for you?"

- Give time expectations—say you'll be back in 20 minutes or that you'll check in at 9 o'clock. If you can't make it, just stick your head in the door and give the patient an update—"I'll be there in five minutes."

- Don't ever tell the patient everything else you have to do or act rushed. Your actions and words must reflect that you have time for them—or their anxiety will increase.

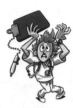

Don't panic: "What do you do when you know the patient wants you to spend more time with him or her—but you just can't." Acknowledge the patient's feelings. The worst thing you can do is to ignore or make light of the patient's request. Use the DESC (describe, explain, state, consequence) model.

D	**Describe** the behavior
E	**Explain** the impact of the behavior
S	**State** the desired outcome
C	**Consequence**—what will happen if the behavior continues? (Cox)

Some people like to memorize the key words that represent this model because it gives them structure:

D	When . . .
E	I feel . . . Because . . .
S	Therefore, I want/need . . .
C	So that . . .

For example:

D	"I know you would like me to stay and talk, and I would like to speak with you as well."
E	"I can't do that right now."
S	"But I want you to know that I will come back as soon as I can, and we will have a chance to speak before lunch."
C	"If you need someone immediately, I can call the chaplain or charge nurse. But if you can wait 30 minutes, I'd love to talk to you."

Tip: Don't ever say or imply that you have something more important to do than helping the patient you are with at that time. Instead, say, "It's really important I help you with that. I can do that in X minutes."

Chapter 6

Dealing with death

Listen up: "Karen paged you. I told her you were in a meeting."

"What did she want?"

"She said the lady in 967 is close to death. No family. Where are you going?"

"To 967."

"Why?"

"Because on our floor, we believe strongly that no one should ever die alone."

Years ago, people were less afraid and more knowledgeable about death than they are today. Family members once bathed their own dead, and wakes were held in family living rooms instead of funeral parlors. People of all ages experienced death on a very visceral level, and death was viewed as a part of the cycle of life.

But today, death is farther out of our reach and exists more in the realm of the unknown. Many new nurses are apprehensive about talking with patients about the issues of death and dying for several reasons. We live in a culture that bombards us with commercial products that postpone aging indefinitely, as if they were a modern-day fountain of youth. In addition, many nurses have never seen anyone die before—and it is human nature to be afraid of the unknown. Not only do we feel unprepared and inexperienced when someone dies, but we are reminded of our own mortality, which can be uncomfortable no matter how old you are.

"Life is pleasant. Death is peaceful. It's the transition that's troublesome."

—Isaac Asimov

Helping to write the final chapter

Think of everyone's life as an incredible story. As wonderful as any book is, there is always a last chapter. As nurses, our primary role is to ensure that the last chapter is:

1. Defined by the patient rather than imposed by the institution or family members

2. Consistent with how they lived their lives (i.e., the theme of their story)

For example, a patient may want to die at home, contact a friend, or be surrounded by their pets (Loughlin). Your role is to help patients to die as they lived.

Think of yourself as helping patients and families navigate a chart—you are the mapmaker in uncharted territory. Patients and family members have no idea what road to go down. They don't even know which questions to ask, let alone what to do. As nurses, it is our job to help patients become aware of their choices and their consequences. A common mistake made by physicians and nurses is that they feel helpless and want to "do something." But hanging an IV, for example, only prolongs death because while the major organs are shutting down, an IV inhibits natural pain-relieving chemicals that are released when the body dehydrates (Dunn). So when a physician asks the family, "You want a feeding tube, don't you?" family members automatically feel the need to agree, not fully understanding that the patient will not improve and that the feeding tube is just buying time.

When dealing with impending death, patients and their families are unprepared for and overwhelmed by the decisions that suddenly present themselves: Ventilator? Code status? Feeding tube? Your role is to help patients and their families formulate the questions and get the answers to facilitate choices. And to do that, you need to be knowledgeable.

Here are some facts you should know:

- Patients with advanced dementia, such as end-stage Alzheimer's disease, will not be helped with the use of artificial feeding tubes and may actually be harmed.

- A time-limited trial can be used to try a treatment for a period of time. If it does not help the patient, then it can be discontinued.

- Dying patients are *much more comfortable* without the use of artificial hydration.

- Permanently unconscious patients can be maintained for years with a feeding tube, but people disagree whether such treatment should on when or whether the tube should be withdrawn.

- The average survival rate for all patients who have CPR attempts is 15.2% (Dunn).

What do I say? What do I do?

When new nurses were asked to name communication situations where they felt uncomfortable, death and dying issues were a common theme. One student said, "I don't have an appropriate response to death. I don't know what to do or say."

Don't panic: First of all, there isn't one. The only response you can give is to be fully present, to be willing to simply stay with the patient and family in their time of grief and fear and not run away. Your main job is to stand witness to the moment of passing so that both patient and family feel your presence, support, and caring. Their hearts will lean against you as if you were a sturdy oak.

End-of-life discussions are often informed by the person's or family's culture, and this may affect with whom an end-of-life conversation may occur (in some cultures it may not be the patient) and what words may or may not be used. The EthnoMed Web site (*www.ethnomed.org*) can be a helpful resource for nurses in increasing their understanding of individual cultures' practices about medical discussions and truth-telling.

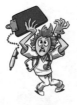

Don't panic: "What do family members want?"

They want to know they have done everything possible and that they respected the choices of their loved one. They want to know the facts: prognosis, possible outcomes, timelines, and what to expect.

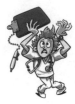

Don't panic: "What do the dying say they appreciate most from a nurse?"

"They appreciate someone who is accepting and who listens, a nurse who is willing to be with them. Often, patients will toss out a little bait to see if you are willing to talk. Don't shut down, brush [it] off, or make a joke. Families often brush their comments off because they can't deal with death, and nurses often don't have the time. Be aware that by throwing out a little comment, the patient is testing the waters to see if it's safe to talk to you."

"Families often deflect their loved one's attempts to engage them in an end-of-life discussion because they do not feel comfortable or prepared to talk about death and dying. Nurses may do the same because they may lack the time and may not feel comfortable responding. Be aware that my throwing out a little comment, the patient may be testing your response to see if it is safe to talk to you."

—Gail Loughlin, RN, Providence Hospice of Seattle

Here are some questions you can ask to help with a difficult time:

- What is most important to you right now?

- What does *comfort* mean to you?

- Is there anything you are concerned or worried about?

- This must be hard. Can I just sit with you for awhile? (Dunn)

- Is there anything I can do for you? Is there anything you need?

- Can I answer any questions for you?

And here are a few tips:

- Be willing to "go there." Be present at this time in the patient's journey.

- Let your patient be your teacher. You don't have to have all the answers.

- Listen. Listen. Listen. Be comfortable with silence.

Nowhere in nursing will you find yourself advocating for a patient's rights more than when a patient is dying, because we live in a culture that believes death is a disease to be conquered instead of a part of the natural cycle of life. Should you need support or clarification on any issues, contact your manager, the hospital ethics committee, or pastoral care. Together, we can all ensure that our patients die with dignity and that the transition is natural and peaceful.

For some extra reading on the topic, check out these books:

- *Hard Choices for Loving People: CPR, Artificial Feeding, Comfort Care and the Patient with a Life-Threatening Illness,* 4th edition, by Hank Dunn

- *Tuesdays with Morrie: An Old Man, a Young Man, and Life's Greatest Lesson,* by Mitch Albom

- *Letting Go: Morrie's Reflections on Living While Dying,* by Morrie Schwartz

- *How We Die: Reflections on Life's Final Chapter,* by Sherwin B. Nuland

Part Two

Even though we're all on the same team, nurses don't always see eye-to-eye. Horizontal hostility and unhealthy workplaces have unfortunately made their marks on the industry. This section will tell you how you can start reversing the trend and get everyone shooting for the same goal.

Chapter 7

Join the club: Assimilation into the nursing culture

> *"The conversation is not about the relationship. The conversation is the relationship."*
>
> —Susan Scott

Communication is a search for our common ground. It's all about connecting. In the end, we all want the same things: to be valued, appreciated, and recognized; to learn and grow; and to belong and be a part of something larger than ourselves. Nurses have their patients' interests at heart. They consistently demonstrate their desire to give the most excellent care possible.

What is the primary motivation for nurse-to-nurse communication? Seldom do I hear nurses having patient care disagreements. Generally, nurses seek validation of their assessments from each other and agree on the patient's plan of care. The primary source of peer conflict is almost always personal—a misunderstanding or a feeling of being hurt, used, betrayed, or put upon. It's always some thorn in our relationship. Communicating with peers, then, is primarily about honoring our feelings.

It is imperative that you take care of your emotions. No one can think straight when they are upset. By its very nature, nursing requires mental dexterity—to calculate, reevaluate, and plan care. The gentle hand that strokes the forehead of a dying patient must also be able to swiftly move to the next room and titrate a dopamine drip. Nurses are often heard saying that their "real education" began when they hit the floor because they learned so much about the magnificent art and science of their profession from each other.

 ## Nurses: In their shoes

> *"Never judge another until you have walked three miles in their moccasins."*
>
> —Indian proverb

Since the average age of today's nurse is 47, most of the nurses you meet on the floor will have been in the profession for more than 20 years. They are tired.

The past 10 years have been especially difficult. As hospitals look for ways to cut costs, senior administrators have cut support to staff nurses—especially in the area of education and the time nurses need to adequately care for their patients (i.e., hours of care). Nurses are dedicated both to providing great patient care and to their hospital's financial survival. They live between a rock *and* a hard place.

They work very hard, but no one sees it—not even the other nurses. Everyone is too busy. Our work, which was always invisible to the patients and doctors, has now become invisible to each other. Nurses feel unappreciated.

Compliments are as rare as a lunar eclipse. A thank-you from a doctor? Same thing. Even the managers who used to notice and value great patient care are overwhelmed and absent. Managers' span of control has increased drastically, so now they often supervise more than 100 employees with no administrative support. They have many additional challenges and responsibilities: implementation of new systems for technology, patient safety, regulatory compliance, recruitment, and retention. You just don't see them around on the floor much these days.

In addition, small talk has decreased, so nurses don't know as much about each other. The conversations that usually bind us—the stories we share about our patients and our lives—are just not taking place. Many nurses now work 12-hour shifts two or three days in a row. Little energy remains for socializing. Even the pace of life at home is faster and stretched to the limit. We don't have the free time we used to. No one has the time.

Even the patients have changed. Sometimes, they are in and out the door so fast that nurses don't have time to learn their names: "742 is crying . . . 744 needs a bedpan . . . " If a patient can urinate, drink, and walk to the bathroom, and his or her pain is controlled, the patient is discharged—even if its 10 o'clock at night. Patients are also physically heavier. Neck and back injuries in nurses have increased dramatically as nurses attempt to lift and turn their obese patients. Nurses who have been working on a unit for over 25 years have no other option but to continue working as a staff nurse until retirement. And patients have more secondary and chronic illnesses, which not only require a lot more medications but also result in more complications. Many nurses burn out because the patients are harder work.

Our caregivers are hurting.

> "The greatest need of the soul is for belonging."
>
> —Thomas Moore

So join the club—or try to . . .

If you went to a foreign country and planned on staying there for a while, you would need to blend into that culture in order to feel accepted. Soon after arriving, you would notice the nation's customs: its peoples' common behaviors, language, mannerisms, and greetings. The "normal" way in which people handle daily conflicts, which topics were acceptable for public discussion, etc., would soon become obvious to you. And to fit in, you too would start acting the same way. This process is called *assimilation*.

The nursing culture is no exception. As a new nurse, you have surely observed some of the norms and behaviors on the unit. These behaviors are very subtle and never written down. It's "just the way we've always done it around here." Because there is nothing more important than belonging, nurses begin acting in a way that they would never consciously choose. Being accepted by the group means everything.

Alarm: "There are many cliques on my unit to which I don't feel like I belong. When I try to join in on a group, they don't make eye contact and walk away at times."

And so the cycle continues. New nurses come to the floor and are treated by the older nurses the same way the older nurses were treated when they were younger. Sometimes, newer nurses even report that their experience is more like a college hazing—like they have to prove their worth in order to belong. This seldom-acknowledged observation about our culture can make even the most basic conversations a challenge. So before learning about nurse-to-nurse communication, you must know *and understand* the culture that you are stepping into.

Alarm: "I remember being a new nurse, and when I would ask a question, the other nurses would ask me a question back instead of answering me. This made me feel like I was always being put on the spot and created more stress when I was just searching for support."

Alarm: The charge nurse always gives new, younger nurses the most challenging patients and does not want to help or mentor. Her attitude is, "She's young and thinks she knows it all"—and the unspoken is, "I'll show her."

Why do nurses *act* that way?

It's human nature. Any group of people who have no power and work in a time-constrained, high-pressure environment with very high stakes—human life—would *act exactly the same way*. Sociologists found that people without power unconsciously take out their frustrations on each other. The key word here is *unconsciously*. This is called *horizontal hostility*.

The history of nursing holds a tremendous amount of clues about our identity and, more specifically, about our lack of power. About 150 years ago, nurses came from the middle or lower class in a predominately male society. To be around men, nursing was portrayed as "God's work." Angels never complain, work tirelessly, and sacrifice everything. Because they are so totally immersed in the culture, nurses do not acknowledge or see these unhealthy behaviors. If only senior nurses realized what they were doing.

This situation, however, is on the mend. Nurses are reclaiming their power in many ways. Nursing leaders are spearheading major initiatives to create a healthy workplace environment. Many organizations are pursuing American Nurses Credentialing Center (ANCC) Magnet® status and practicing shared governance—both of which give power back to nurses. The ANCC, an affiliate of the American Nurses Association, awards Magnet status to hospitals after they exemplify a level of excellence and quality in their nursing. Shared governance is an innovative model that gives staff nurses control over their practice at the bedside as well as influence over administrative areas.

Education has expanded to include classes in communication and conflict-management skills, and new nurses are coming into the profession armed with a brand-new set of communication skills. You are entering nursing at the beginning of a communication revolution. And really, it will be up to you to help it take root.

Chapter 8

Changing history: We need you!

Only fresh eyes can help us see some of the unhealthy behaviors in nursing—the rest of us have lived with them for so long, we think it's normal. We desperately need new nurses to help us heal from the insidious behaviors that are hurting our profession. New nurses are in a pivotal position. They can change history by refusing to tolerate horizontal hostility. They can help us see that picking on a new nurse is not normal!

Here's an example:

Martha Griffin prepared her students for the culture they were going to walk into. She noted that it was not the verbal communication that new nurses were having a problem with, but rather the nonverbal responses of the nurses that were precepting her student nurses. Students were puzzled by the innuendos, raised eyebrows, and facial expressions that were clearly negative but didn't actually match the words the nurses were saying (Griffin).

NEWS FLASH! THIS JUST IN!

Twenty-six special agent nurses quietly infiltrated a hospital a year ago disguised as ordinary nurses. Armed with verbal counter-attack tactics, they apparently wiped out the enemy's entire arsenal of non-verbal weaponry on the first day. The planned maneuvering began when a senior nurse smirked and rolled her eyes at the end of the shift. One of "The 26" stopped her midsarcasm with the words, "Excuse me, but even though you said I did great today, I noticed you rolled your eyes just now. If there is something that you want to say, you can say it to me directly." The senior nurse's jaw dropped. An eerie silence came over the nurses' station. Who were "The 26?" And who was this brave nurse who could end a century-old pattern of abuse in just two sentences?

Witnesses say that things just haven't been the same since that fateful day. New nurses are reveling in their first year as senior nurses support them in every way they possibly can, happily passing on their love of nursing to a new generation.

It's not that the older nurses didn't try to put the new nurses down, but rather the students knew *what to expect* and had practiced *how to respond*. Because of this, they were able to stop the cycle of horizontal hostility. You can, too. By demonstrating similar responses, you will have a tremendous influence in creating a healthier workplace environment. We need you. Say what you see. Call a spade a spade.

 Tip: Always speak your truth.

The following table will show you how to react when faced with certain instances of horizontal hostility:

Responses to horizontal hostility

SIDE 1

Nonverbal innuendo (raising of eyebrows, face-making).
- I sense (I see from your facial expression) that there may be something you wanted to say to me. It's okay to speak directly to me.

Verbal affront (covert or overt, snide remarks, lack of openness, abrupt responses).
- The individuals I learn the most from are clearer in their directions and feedback. Is there some way we can structure this type of situation?

Undermining activities (turning away, being unavailable).
- When something happens that is "different" or "contrary" to what I thought or understood, it leaves me with questions. Help me understand how this situation may have happened.

Withholding information (practice or patient).
- It is my understanding that there was (is) more information available regarding the situation, and I believe if I had known that (more), it would (will) affect how I learn.

Sabotage (deliberately setting up a negative situation).
- There is more to this situation than meets the eye. Could "you and I" (whatever, whoever) meet in private and explore what happened?

Responses to horizontal hostility (cont.)

SIDE 2

Infighting (bickering with peers). Nothing is more unprofessional than a contentious discussion in a nonprivate place. Always avoid.
- This is not the time or the place. Please stop (physically walk away or move to a neutral spot).

Scapegoating (attributing all that goes wrong to one individual). Rarely is one individual, one incident, or one situation the cause for all that goes wrong. Scapegoating is an easy route to travel, but it rarely solves problems.
- I don't think that's the right connection.

Backstabbing (complaining to others about an individual and not speaking directly to that individual).
- I don't feel right talking about him/her/the situation when I wasn't there or don't know the facts. Have you spoken to him/her?

Failure to respect privacy.
- It bothers me to talk about that without his/her/their permission.
- I only overheard that. It shouldn't be repeated.

Broken confidences.
- Wasn't that said in confidence?
- That sounds like information that should remain confidential.
- He/she asked me to keep that confidential.

It's all about (communication) style

The most common communication style in nursing is passive-aggressive: expressing negative feelings in an unassertive way. This means communicating with other nurses can often be a challenge. Nurses typically don't communicate directly with the person with whom they have a problem, but rather act aggressively toward them through a backdoor approach.

Alarm: Nurses appear annoyed or bothered with the presence of a nursing student, yet are not willing to discuss or resolve issues.

Silence is not always golden

There is nothing in our nursing history that has ever encouraged nurses to speak up. From a spiritual perspective, to talk about "God's work" would be self-aggrandizing. From the perspective of a male-dominated society, a physician could simply walk into administration and have any nurse whom he disliked fired on the spot. Just try saying what you think in that kind of environment. Historically, nurses are silent.

When was the last time you heard a nurse quoted as an expert on the radio or television? Two prominent journalists found that, as the largest healthcare profession, nursing is grossly underrepresented in the media (Buresh). And when it is represented, our work is never adequately or correctly portrayed. Shows like *Grey's Anatomy* flaunt soap opera relationships among residents, leaving nursing, once again, invisible. It is difficult for nurses to speak up when even the characters on a pretend sitcom or drama are invisible and silent.

Strong imprints form early in life. Nurses' personal histories can also affect how they interact with coworkers. For example, a nurse's family may have dealt with a parent's substance abuse when he or she was young. As a child, the future nurse's learned experience was to tiptoe around the truth, avoiding conflict at any cost. Telling the truth was not psychologically safe. He or she learned to survive by "not rocking the boat."

In addition, for many years, there was no formal way to evaluate a nurse's care. No one ever asked a nurse for his or her opinion about the care another nurse provided. Because there was no constructive way to criticize, nurses expressed their views in a destructive way. Peer evaluations are now turning this around and giving nurses a constructive way to receive feedback.

Communication without words

Nurses talk, just not with their mouths.

Because nurses could not speak up, they became experts on expressing themselves nonverbally. Expression is a basic human need. If there were a medal for the best use of facial features to express what you *really* wanted to say but couldn't, nursing would win hands down.

Tip: Always, *always* respond to the *nonverbal message*.

The vast majority of nursing communication is nonverbal. Likewise, it's the covert or hidden behaviors that are most hurtful because the communication is unclear and left to your interpretation. This uncertainty creates anxiety. Then, we jump to the worst conclusion without checking out the behavior.

The following list will give you a good idea of some common hostile behaviors—both hidden and obvious. *Any* of the following behaviors are unacceptable:

- **Covert:** unfair assignments, sarcasm, eye-rolling, ignoring, making faces behind someone's back, refusing to help, sighing, whining, refusing to work with someone, sabotage, isolation, exclusion, fabrication, etc.

- **Overt:** name calling, bickering, fault-finding, backstabbing, criticism, intimidation, gossip, shouting, blaming, using put-downs, raising eyebrows, etc.

So, in conclusion . . .

In the land of nursing, the culture is passive-aggressive and the predominant language is nonverbal. Now you know nurse-speak.

Chapter 9

Defining your boundaries

When should you speak and when should you be silent? What conversations should you engage in and which ones should you let slide? Are you taking something too personally and being too sensitive, or is another nurse attacking your integrity? Nurse-to-nurse communication must sit within some framework. The first step is to define your boundaries.

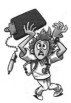

Don't panic: "I don't know how to handle comments made in public to other nurses at the nurses' station that undermine me as a nurse."

Check out the professional behaviors listed by Martha Griffin in the table on the next page. They provide an excellent framework for professional relationships, and therefore for communication standards between peers. The common denominator here is respect—for self and others. Take a moment to read through the list. Do these tenets of professional behavior match your belief system?

Professional behaviors

- Accept one's fair share of the workload.
- Respect the privacy of others.
- Be cooperative with regard to the shared physical working conditions (e.g., light, temperature, noise).
- Be willing to help when requested.
- Keep confidences.
- Work cooperatively despite feelings of dislike.
- Don't denigrate to superiors (e.g., speak negatively about, have a pet name for).
- Do address coworkers by their first name, and ask for help and advice when necessary.
- Look coworkers in the eye when having a conversation.
- Don't be overly inquisitive about each others' lives.
- Do repay debts, favors, and compliments, no matter how small.
- Don't engage in conversation about a coworker with another coworker.
- Stand-up for the "absent member" in a conversation when he/she is not present.
- Don't criticize publicly.

Reprinted with permission from SLACK Incorporated: Griffin, M. (2004). Teaching cognitive rehearsal as a shield for lateral violence: An intervention for newly licensed nurses. *The Journal of Continuing Education in Nursing*, 35 (6), 257-263.

Having a code of conduct sets a clear picture of your own personal boundary line. Any step across this line requires communication—even if it's something as subtle as eye-rolling. *Any* actions or words that make you feel less than the capable and caring nurse you are demands communication. Now you know when to walk away (when one nurse is slamming another face-to-face) and when to engage (defending a nurse who is not present). Every time someone crosses that line and you do not communicate its effect, you lose a little more self-esteem—and by your silence, you endorse the behavior.

Gossip be gone!

> *"When someone dumps their toxic feelings on us . . . they activate in us circuitry for those very same distressing emotions. Their act has powerful neurological consequences: Emotions are contagious."*
>
> —Daniel Goleman, *Social Intelligence*

Bullies and people who make others' lives miserable exist in every profession. Gossip is toxic. It is a lethal poison that kills the morale of an entire unit. Underneath the storytelling is one cold, hard fact that no one says out loud: *"If this person is gossiping about another person, he or she could be talking about me, too."* The workplace then becomes a dangerous place where it is not safe to express yourself for fear of judgment or retaliation.

Here are some tips to help you keep your workplace healthy:

- No discussion concerning another person can take place if that person isn't present.

- All issues must pertain to a behavior that threatens the mission of the organization, including patient safety and professional values.

- If a person has an issue with another person, he or she must privately and directly discuss the issue with the other person.

- All personnel must enforce the policy. Gossip and destructive social behaviors must be addressed by everyone in the environment. (Ramos)

 Listen up: Sam was one of the most cheerful and positive nurses on the unit. She was always offering to help other nurses and volunteering to pick up extra shifts when the unit was short. One day, after a workshop, she came to my office and said, "I had no idea I was contributing to horizontal hostility. I never say anything bad about someone, but I don't walk away when nurses are slamming another nurse who isn't there either. I'll never do that again."

What do I do?

Here are some tips on what to do when nurses around you start putting another nurse down:

- Walk away immediately

- State that you don't want someone talking about you when you're not around, so you're not going to do it to others

- State that it's part of the professional code not to speak about someone when he or she is not present

- Remind the others that you have zero tolerance for hostility on the unit

Chapter 10

Where the rubber meets the road... *How* do I do this again?

You're off to a great start! Understanding the nursing culture and communication style of nurses already puts you in a powerful position (because many nurses themselves don't acknowledge hostility and passive-aggressiveness). Understanding where your peers are coming from is critical. And awareness of your personal boundary line allows you to identify when someone has stepped over it—the moment you *must* say something. This honor code of communication will increase your sense of self-esteem and confidence tremendously, while role modeling the behaviors that make a healthy work environment. Two other skills are critical to great peer communication:

- Knowing your own story

- Knowing your conflict style

Knowing your story

In a counseling workshop I attended years ago, I learned some very important lessons that have helped tremendously:

- You can't control what people do or say, you can only control *your response.*

- There are only two possible actions: You react or you respond.

- When you react, it's always from an emotional level. Emotions will override thoughts every time.

Eruptions and reactions

When you react, when feelings unexpectedly erupt like lava out of a volcano, it is always because something about this conversation has triggered an emotional memory from the past. This is a huge clue. STOP. *Big red flag!* You are taking emotional baggage on this conversation trip. Take a moment to acknowledge the emotions before you proceed any further in the conversation. If a nurse wants to have a conversation immediately, ask for some time to process and digest the emotions you are feeling.

Listen up: Kate and Michelle had been ignoring each other all day. Everyone on the floor could feel the tension. When the manager found out about the hard feelings between the two, she insisted on a crucial conversation at the end of the shift in her office.

But as soon as Kate sat down she said, "I don't want to do this. Do we have to do this today?"

When the manager said, "Yes," tears immediately started rolling down Kate's face.

"What is it?" asked the manager.

"Nothing," Kate said, "just memories of my alcoholic father . . . I'll be okay."

In this situation, Kate made the connection on the spot. Because of this, she was able to continue the conversation—even after the manager then gave her another opportunity to postpone. For Kate, any type of confrontation brought up powerful memories. More often, however, processing emotions takes time.

When you see people react emotionally—displaying anger, hurt, or rage— know that this is linked to one of their past experiences and that they will have a *very significant life story attached to the situation.* You could say, "It looks like this is a difficult conversation for you right now. I really want to talk with you, but let's do this tomorrow." Or you could be empathetic if you sincerely want to hear about the person's experience and say, "You seem upset. Is there anything I can do for you?

60

Tip: Strong emotional reactions are tied to past experiences.

Spell confidence with DESC

When you *respond* to a stimulus, you are in the present moment. Listening is critical. The outcome is not preplanned; the genuine interest is in connecting with another human being. From this place, you can use the DESC model (mentioned in Chapter 5) to "boost your confidence for communicating in a new way . . . It's a great way to get your thoughts in order" (Cox).

Let's apply the model now to answer the following questions frequently asked by new nurses.

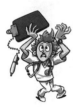

Don't panic: "How do I talk to an experienced nurse when she makes it obvious in many ways that she has no time, patience, or empathy for my concerns?"

D	"I noticed today that you seemed bothered by my questions, and I felt in the way."
E	"I understand you have a heavy workload, but when you ignore me, I feel terrible. I feel unimportant and get the message that you wish I wasn't here."
S	"I need to find some way or some time when I can connect with you. I want to learn and be the best nurse I can be."
C	"If you continue to ignore me and act like I am in the way, I can't stay. I love nursing, but I simply can't learn in this environment."

A closer look at DESC

Feedback Formula	Rational	DESC Model (Intent/impact)	Rational
Facts First	Lead with the facts! Observable, less likely to cause defensiveness, facts are not personal. Facts are seen and heard. Verifiable by others.	Describe the situation	Describe using facts, orient the person to the issue you are discussing with them.
Story Second	Your story is your impression, your interpretation of the facts. Share what the facts meant to you. Your story usually has some emotion attached to it, the facts have caused you to "feel" something. Share your story.	Explain what this means to you	Let the person know the impact of the situation. Tell them how you "see it." This tells them why you are talking to them . . . it is having an impact on you. Share that.
Pause, Pause, Pause	Pausing allows the other person a minute to assimilate what they have just heard. It also prevents you from overwhelming the person and from speaking too fast.	Pause, Pause, Pause	Pausing allows the other person a minute to assimilate what they have just heard. It also prevents you from overwhelming the person and speaking too fast.
Check for understanding	Asking, "How do you see it?" or "Do you see it differently?" invites dialogue. This step is about clarifying the situation you are giving feedback about.	State what you want instead	Discuss behavior you DO want. Be descriptive. Using the affirmative approach helps the other person know what they should do and minimizes defensiveness by not focusing on what is wrong. This step re-frames the situation; "This is what I do want from you." The positive approach can make it easier for the other person to agree with you. It helps them save face.
		Consequences: describe the consequences that will naturally occur if the situation continues. (Motivation is different for each person. Try to describe consequences that matter to this person.)	Describe the impact if the person does not meet the expectation you just "stated." Consequences usually have an impact on 3 levels: Individual: "What is in it for me?" What pain or pleasure is attached to this situation? Outline the benefit to them associated with complying. Social: Impact to others, to the team. What praise or pressure from others might be a consequence? Work environment: Standards, policies, rules, "carrots and sticks" associated with this situation. Progressive Corrective Action is an example of a work consequence/impact.

Source: Adapted from Sharon Cox's DESC model. Courtesy of Anastasia Hartog, Employee Learning, Swedish Medical Center, Seattle.

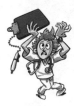

Don't panic: "What do you say after you hear that someone has been backstabbing you?"

D "I'd like to talk with you in private. I heard from another nurse that you said I didn't know what I was doing, that I would never be a good nurse."

E "When I hear that someone has been saying things about me and I don't know why, or even what situation it pertains to, I feel sabotaged and set up to fail."

S "I want to be a good nurse, and I can't do that without your honest feedback and support. Can you say what you feel and think directly to me in private?"

C "Without that support, I am sure to fail. I will have to find another place to work, even though this is the specialty I had chosen."

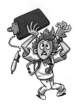

Don't panic: "I work with someone who is always making negative comments. What can I say?"

D "Can I talk to you in private for just a moment? When you came onto the floor at the beginning of the shift and discovered that you had to float, I heard you make some really negative comments. You did it last week, too."

E "I understand that everyone has bad days and that we all need to vent sometimes, but your comments are really depressing for me."

S "I need you to understand that your words have a big influence on my mood."

C "If I have to listen to this every day, I'm concerned this negativity will really affect my morale and my health."

One nurse mentioned to me that he liked to add another **D** to this model for doable. He always ends with an open-ended question, such as "Will this work for you?" or "Is this doable?" In this way, he is actively seeking cooperation and asking for confirmation that what he said was reasonable.

Don't panic: "How do you preserve a friendship, and speak your truth at the same time? I don't want to lose a good friend."

D "I know you and I are good friends, and because of that I have put off this conversation many times."

E "I've followed you three times last week, and each time the meds for a patient were not charted. I was afraid to say something because I didn't want work to affect or jeopardize our friendship, which I really value."

S   "Is there some way that I can let you know about a problem when I see it and you can realize that I am not picking on you? Maybe put a note on your locker?"

C   "Keeping this to myself would be hurtful to our friendship."

D   "Would this work for you?"

 Listen up: Charlie had just come out of report when one of his evening nurses abruptly turned her back and stormed away. "I wonder why she is so mad. I made out a fair assignment," he thought.

A half hour later, Charlie saw the nurse in the hall charting, and he approached her cautiously. "Tammy, I was wondering if I said or did something to offend you in report. You seemed so angry when you turned away at the doorway so abruptly."

"Goodness, no," Tammy said. "Don't you remember from report that one of my postop patients' blood pressure was dangerously low? I just wanted to get to his room quickly to make sure he was all right."

Charlie was trying out his new communication skills. Normally, he would have been extremely reluctant to approach Tammy, who had a powerful personality. Using the DESC model, he described how he felt and named the behavior without putting Tammy in the defensive position.

Here are some sources of interpersonal conflict in the clinical area:

- Being asked to do something you know would be irresponsible or unsafe
- Having your feelings or opinions ridiculed or discounted
- Being pressured to give more time or attention than you are able to give
- Being asked to give more information than you feel comfortable sharing
- Maintaining a sense of self in the face of hostility or sexual harassment

  (Arnold, Boggs)

Knowing your conflict style

Conflict isn't a bad thing. It is not to be avoided at all costs, or pursued to the point of hounding. Look at conflict as a doorway, a rare opportunity to enter another person's world. Everyone enters each conversation from the point of view of his or her own life experiences. Your responsibility in conflict is to speak your truth and listen to others' truths.

People respond to conflict differently. We respond based on our values. What do you value? Every one of us has a primary conflict style and a default style. Knowing your style is extremely helpful, especially in unexpected conflicts—and most conflicts are unexpected. For example, if you realize that you accommodate all the time, you may start to feel ineffective and your self-esteem will falter because you don't accomplish your goal. If you use an avoidance style, you would really have to work hard to speak up to a peer who is upset.

A variety of conflict styles

Here are some different conflict styles. Everyone has a primary style that they use most of the time and a secondary style that they can default to if the primary is ineffective. Decide which ones describe you best:

Collaborative   You value the relationships and the goal that needs to be accomplished.

Compromise   You believe you must give a little to get a little.

Accommodation   You believe you should relinquish your goals to maintain a relationship.

Forcing   You value the task at hand—the goal—as most important.

Avoidance   Neither the goal nor the relationship are worth the conflict.

My primary conflict style is _____.

Sometimes I default to _____.

Chapter 11

Communication cheat sheet

Tools and techniques for you to use

Communication is more than just one person talking to another person.
There are strategies and methods you can use to get the most out of your
interactions. Let's outline them now.

Listen

We talk at 125-250 words per minute, listen at 450–900 words per minute,
but can think at up to 3,000 words per minute. So when someone is talking,
we have plenty of extra time on our hands. How do we spend this time?
Usually, we are planning our next response.

Real listening is a skill that must be practiced. It is about staying in a receiving space so you can really understand what someone is saying. Next time
you have a conversation, pay special attention to how many times your
mind wanders.

Silence

If you are having trouble in a conversation, there is another option. Silence.
The more emotionally loaded the subject, the more silence is required. Here
are some signs that silence is needed:

- Interrupting by talking over someone else

- Responding quickly with little or no thought

- Formulating your own response while someone is talking

- Using a break in the conversation to create a distraction by changing topics

- Talking in circles, meaning nothing new emerges (Scott)

Be authentic

If you don't understand what someone is saying, ask the person to state it in another way. *Don't ever pretend* you know what someone is talking about if you don't—it's a waste of time and energy for both of you. For any meaningful conversation to occur, you have to be your genuine self at all times. Your willingness to be yourself in a conversation reflects your willingness to be yourself in relationship with your peers.

Slow down

If you are not sure whether you understand the other person, stop and paraphrase. "Are you saying . . . ?" or "What I hear you saying is . . . Is that right?" Not only does this clear things up for you, but it also validates what the other person is saying and lets him or her know that you understand.

Prepare

Assess your readiness to be in the conversation. It's your right to ask to have the conversation at another time. If you can't be fully present because something else is on your mind, reschedule. If this is going to be a difficult or emotional conversation for you, practice. Use the DESC model to jot down your thoughts. Ask yourself:

- What is the purpose/goal of this conversation?

- What do I need?

- What outcome do I want?

- Are my intentions sincere?

- What is my story? Do I have any emotional "baggage" about this issue?

Be creative

There are lots of ways to get a message across!

 Listen up: Kari knew this was going to be difficult. She really liked Shawna, but working with Shawna drove her crazy. When Shawna came up to the nurses' station, it was always mass confusion. She talked and moved constantly. Kari had put off giving her feedback all week, but today they planned to have lunch together. Kari was nervous, but she had given this conversation a lot of thought.

"Have you ever noticed that people remind you of animals?" asked Kari.

"What do you mean?" asked Shawna.

"Well, you know Terri and how meek and quiet she is. What does she remind you of?"

"A deer," said Shawna.

"That's what I thought! And what about Gus? What do his movements remind you of? He has such a presence."

"A rhino," said Shawna, getting into the game.

"And what about me? What animal do my movements remind you of?"

"Hmm . . . Never thought about it that way," said Shawna. "I guess you would be an owl or an eagle because you always see what's going on."

"And what about you?" asked Kari.

Shawna was quiet. Kari was comfortable with the silence.

"I guess I'm more like that roadrunner bird."

More silence. Then Kari said thoughtfully, "Sometimes it's hard for the owl to be around the roadrunner energy all day long."

Shawna got it. She had never stopped to think about how her racing around affected others, and the conversation helped her to see how her kinetic energy level affected others. Kari achieved her goal: raising Shawna's level of awareness while maintaining her sense of self-esteem.

Don't preload

Assuming . . . guessing . . . supposing . . . judging . . . is all about you. They are all signs that you made up your own story without the need to confirm with another person. When you already have your mind made up, it's not a conversation at all. Leave the judge and jury at home and meet on the hilltop, human to human.

Intention is everything

Be aware of your true motive.

Listen up: Danny wanted advice on how to give constructive feedback to a peer—especially when it was just his opinion that a peer should do things differently. The more Danny talked, the more it became obvious that what Danny really wanted was to prove he was a better nurse. The tone underneath his words betrayed his true motive. No wonder these conversations ended in disaster!

Tip: Tone of voice will always communicate your true motive.

Chapter 12

Trouble spots . . . Ouch!

> "The most valuable thing any of us can do is find a way to say the things that can't be said."
>
> —Susan Scott, *Fierce Conversations*

As nurses, we make every attempt to see the whole person. We are taught to look with compassion at the spiritual, emotional, psychological, and physical pieces of information presented by the patient and combine them with our physical assessment to paint the "big picture." Healing has many forms. Often, helping patients find meaning in their experience is more healing to the patient than any medication or treatment. This is the essence of holistic nursing.

What happens if we use that same holistic focus to look at communication with our peers? How can we find meaning in our everyday communication when we are dealing with so many different personalities from different cultures, all with their own stories?

To paraphrase Einstein, "The belief in our separateness is an optical delusion." Negative people express a group's disappointments; difficult nurses express the group's problems; aloof nurses express the group's disillusionment; and angry nurses express the group's pain. We need to adopt a new belief system that acts as the foundation for all communication, one that articulates our dependence on and compassion for each other. What would these new beliefs be?

- We are all in this together

- We are only as strong as our weakest link

- Everyone has something special to offer—if you can't see it, look harder

- Our greatest strength is in the relationships we have with each other

- Compassion and kindness go a lot further than judgment and blame

- Nobody is perfect

- Everyone has his or her own story—don't make one up before listening to that person's

- If you have a problem with someone, speak to that person in private

- Negativity poisons the workplace to the point that it can make us physically sick

- We are all responsible for creating a positive workspace—by our verbal or nonverbal communications

But here is *my* problem . . .

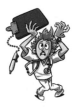

Don't panic: "I don't understand difficult nurses. What makes them think they can treat people so rudely?"

The answer: Because no one stops them. No one confronts these nurses about their behavior because these people usually have very strong personalities (e.g., he or she is the alpha dog in the pack). And the main reason people don't stop them is because nurses take the offense so personally. When we are hurt or wounded, *our natural instinct is to back off.* Nurses are by nature sensitive people—we have to be in order to be sensitive to our patients' needs. But it's important to realize that we are also extremely sensitive to each other.

Remember:

- Don't tolerate this behavior from anyone

- Don't take it personally

- Always speak your truth

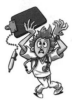

Don't panic: "I don't know how to even begin handling experienced, jaded nurses. Where do you start?"

Answer: At the truth. Use the DESC model to describe specifically how jaded nurses' behavior affects you. People are a result of their experiences, and these apathetic nurses are wounded nurses who have put up a front so they can't be hurt again. It is almost always a defense or coping mechanism. Can you see beyond the front?

- Ask about their first experience as a nurse. Be curious.

- Ask them to share their story. Care.

- Ask for their help. There is no textbook in the world that could adequately capture the wealth of knowledge of even one experienced nurse.

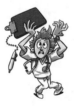

Don't panic: "How do you handle unfair assignments? The hardest thing for me is an unfair assignment (sepsis, encephalitis, and one new spinal cord injury). The charge nurse asked if I needed any help, and I told her specifically that I needed a patient escorted to an appointment. She then lectured me that I needed to learn how to prioritize my time better. I didn't have lunch or a break all shift. The spinal cord injury patient was crying and upset and I couldn't spend any time with him to meet his emotional needs."

Often, new nurses hesitate to speak up about an unfair assignment because they question their own competence. They are unsure about whether it is their lack of experience that makes the assignment so difficult, and they want to demonstrate that they are indeed competent. If they speak up, the fear is that they will be perceived as whining and not pulling their fair share.

Tip: Here's a reality check: If you feel overwhelmed, then you are overwhelmed. Trust yourself. Validate and communicate your perceptions. The key to communicating about unfair assignments is speaking up. After a difficult shift, briefly jot down the key stressors that captured so much of your physical and emotional attention. Share them with the charge nurse in private *the next day you work*. If this becomes a consistent pattern, speak to your educator or manager.

In the situations that I have investigated in which nurses thought an assignment was unfair, the charge nurse who made the assignment was truly unaware of the complications that arose during the shift. The charge nurse does not have a crystal ball that can predict which patients will be challenging. On one occasion, the charge nurse had not worked for a week and was not familiar enough with the patients to make an equitable assignment.

Always ask for help from the charge nurse when you need it. Good nurses need help—and good charge nurses truly want their new nurses to succeed and feel supported.

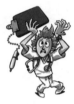

Don't panic: "How do I deal with nurses who complain all the time?"

Ask them for a solution. Some nurses get a lot of attention by constantly whining. Turn the discussion around and refocus the conversation to the solution:

1. Acknowledge the problem

2. Review the details

3. Brainstorm for solutions

Make sure as much energy goes into solving the problem as goes into presenting the problem. Don't listen to the same complaint repeatedly. If this situation is dragging one nurse down, it is probably bothering others as well and deserves consideration.

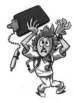

Don't panic: "I don't know what to do when I find mistakes other nurses have made. I don't want to let errors slide, but at the same time, I don't want my peers to think I am picking on them—or that I think I am better than them."

The goal is to create an environment where everyone on the team realizes they are human beings—and human beings will never be perfect. We all make mistakes. That is why we need each other and why working as a team is so important. That is the aspiration.

The reality, however, is that we have operated for years in an environment where people were punished or looked down upon for making errors. Such negative energy around mistakes has decreased our sense of self-esteem. Therefore, many nurses find it hard to receive feedback and even harder to give feedback directly to the person involved. The culture is changing, however, and your response to mistakes in the workplace is critical to creating a safer environment for your patients.

Don't leave notes on lockers or send e-mails regarding mistakes—it's too sensitive an issue. You can't reveal your intention (tone of voice) unless the exchange is face to face. All too often written notes feel like an attack. Always speak to a peer about mistakes face to face.

Tip: If you judge the error to be significant, say something *every time*. For example, "I followed you yesterday, and I thought you might want to know that there were no I&Os charted for Mr. Wilson even though the order was strict I&Os due to his cardiac heart failure."

Tip: If the error is insignificant, let it slide once or twice. But if you notice a pattern, you should say something. For example, "I followed you last week, and every day there was a section uncharted in the nurses' notes. I wanted to tell you because I knew if I didn't say something, you would have never known about it."

Tip: What if you are at the receiving end of the line? Your response is just as crucial in building a culture of safety. Even the smallest of mistakes can be a part of the chain of events that produces a sentinel event. "Thank you for telling me. I'll check my charting before I leave for the day to set up a double check. Please let me know if you notice it again."

Don't panic: "There is another nurse on our floor from another country who thinks she knows it all. Her arrogance bothers me, but maybe it's a cultural thing?"

> *"The world in which you were born is just one model of reality. Other cultures are not failed attempts at being you; they are unique manifestations of the human spirit."*
>
> —Wade Davis

Context is critical. Perhaps, in this case, in the nurse's country of origin women had to struggle extremely hard to prove their intelligence. Every culture has a unique story. Assume that every nurse is trying to do his or her clinical best until proven otherwise.

If it really bothers you, it's time for a "crucial conversation"—but not from a point of judgment. (After all, it's your problem, not hers.) You could use the DESC model and give very specific examples of the behavior and your perceptions/feelings. Either you will walk away with keener insight and respect for your peer's journey into a new country, or your peer will walk away with keener insight into how he or she is coming across in a foreign culture. What's the goal? It is not to force someone to change; it is to be on the same wavelength so you can work together with mutual respect as team members.

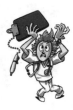

Don't panic: "I start sweating just at the thought of approaching someone with a difficult topic."

Take several long deep breaths or shrug your shoulders. Both of these actions have been known to stop the cascade of physical symptoms that happen when you feel yourself getting into the "flight or fright" mode.

> *"How we lead our days is how we lead our lives."*
>
> —Anne Dillard

A healthy communication list

In search of better nurse-to-nurse communication? Feel free to pass this list along:

- Compliment someone *every day*. It's not just about saying something nice, it's about the fact that you noticed, that you paid attention to a peer's unique talent.

- Speak your truth. Don't harbor resentments. The price is too high. Find the courage to say what is on your mind. Take care of your emotional self.

- Don't tolerate negativity. You can catch negative emotions just as easily as you can catch a cold—and a negativity virus will infect the whole floor like gangrene.

- A simple "thank you" goes a long way. Stop to thank your nursing assistant or another nurse who helped you out during the shift.

- Take care of your physical self. Take meal breaks and bring snacks. Stay as hydrated as an athlete.

Part Three

Sometimes it might feel like nurses and physicians are from two different planets. From the ones that bark orders to ones that are downright negative, docs can be pretty intimidating. This section will help you to level the playing field and get on the same wavelength. Soon, working together will be out of this world!

Chapter 13

Nurses are from Venus, doctors are from Mars

 Alarm: Why don't MDs respect the assessments and recommendations from the bedside RN?

The curriculum for physicians and the curriculum for nurses are completely independent of each other. At no point in their education do the two ever meet. Therefore, physicians graduate without an understanding of the nurse's role. Physicians simply do not have a realistic picture of the tasks and responsibilities facing nurses today. Yet nurses work with physicians more than any other member of the healthcare team.

Knowledge isn't the only thing physicians learn in med school. During their educational process, physicians adopt behaviors (e.g., a dominating tone of voice or a particular way of treating nurses) from their mentors. Some of these behaviors can be intimidating and have caused, among other things, seasoned nurses to remain silent about their patient care concerns or to fail to question a doctor's order. **Don't take physicians' behaviors personally.**

Doctors: In their shoes

> "Never judge another until you have walked three miles in their moccasins."
>
> —Indian proverb

Physician morale has decreased significantly over the past 10 years, with the most affected group being doctors between the ages of 50 and 60. Physicians work harder than ever before, yet their profit margins are shrinking due to decreased reimbursements and escalating malpractice insurance costs. Some are still paying off tremendously high college loans. Reimbursement rates for medical care are cut back every year, and insurance companies index their reimbursements accordingly. More office staff is needed to get insurance approval.

Studies show that with every additional year of medical school, physicians' empathy decreases. As residents, most physicians worked more than 100 hours in a single week. With minds that worked like ACLS flow charts in a time-constrained environment, they simply didn't have time to process emotions. Feelings take time. In addition, doctors were taught to focus only on the clinical signs and symptoms, which tends to obscure the emotional and psychological needs of patients. Today, several universities are trying to improve physicians' empathy by adding classes in narrative medicine, journaling, and spirituality.

Physician autonomy is threatened as nurse practitioners replace many of the jobs that only physicians used to do. Gone are the days of Marcus Welby with the caduceus sign on every physician's license plate and free parking—we now live in a litigious society. The "culture code" for physicians in our society is that they should be heroes—and if they can't save us from death or disease, well then they must be negligent (Rapaille).

Because of access to the Internet, patients come into their doctors' offices telling them what to do, and so doctors spend a great deal of time discussing the volumes of Internet information found by their patients. A tremendous amount of publicly available data has replaced a long-held, sacred trust. In addition, technology is advancing so rapidly that doctors need to constantly educate themselves on new techniques, equipment, or procedures while putting in more hours than they did 10 years ago.

Our medicine men—and women—are hurting.

Even though studies show that 92.5% of nurses have witnessed disruptive behavior (Rosenstein), it's really caused by a very small percentage of doctors—less than 10%. Don't let one bad experience influence your perception of the collegial relationship you can have with a physician. In addition, med school graduating classes are now more than 50% female, so the demographics are changing.

The nursing code of conduct

Research shows there is a direct correlation between the relationship a physician and nurse have and the mortality rate of their patients (Baggs). The bottom line: Negative relationships equal negative outcomes for patients. By virtue of our code of conduct, we should do *everything in our power* to create the collegial relationships associated with positive outcomes for our patients. What's in *"your* power?"

Your response!

Communication is all about the relationship. Relationships with physicians have been classified into five major categories. As the categories move from top to bottom, the physician retains more power. That's why it takes a lot of courage to deal with negative behaviors successfully—the physicians act out this power in dominant behaviors, which makes it very difficult to approach them.

Rungs on the nurse-physician relationship ladder

- **Collegial:** The physician respects you as an equal, asks for, and listens to your advice.
- **Collaborative:** The physician listens, but both of you know he has the last word.
- **Teacher-student:** The relationship focuses on teaching and learning—strictly scholastic.
- **Neutral:** What relationship?
- **Negative:** You'll do anything to avoid him or her; the physician is disruptive and hurtful.

What are some of the ways physicians maintain their dominance? The majority of these behaviors are nonverbal:

- Poor eye contact or raised eyebrows

- Never bothering to learn your name

- Ignoring you

- Giving one-word answers

- Using a sarcastic tone of voice

- Body language that says, "I am better than you"

- Eyes that say, "You are bothering me"

Acknowledging this power difference is the *first step* in learning to communicate with physicians, because the vast majority of all communication is nonverbal. As new nurses, sometimes we just can't put our finger on why we hesitate to approach a physician. You may need to remind yourself that these are *learned behaviors* and not to take them personally.

 Alarm: "I didn't expect the physician to become a little defensive after I politely asked why my patient is receiving a drug that must be used with caution in patients with sulfa allergies—and my patient had a sulfa allergy. I clearly was seeking an explanation, not proof of the provider's competence."

The *second step* is to always direct (or redirect) the focus of the conversation to both your and the physician's common goal: the best possible outcome for the patient.

Listen up: Sally dreaded calling the physician's assistant. During morning rounds, he had told her that the patient's discharge prescriptions were in the chart—but she couldn't find them anywhere. Sally searched the floor, asking the charge nurse to help as the patient kept ringing the call light to be discharged home. Finally, she called the physician's assistant who yelled into the phone, "I told you that I put them in the chart, and I am not writing them out again for you!"

"Please stop," Sally said. "The prescriptions are not for me. They are for our patient, whom I am trying to help go home. I am sending someone over to your office to pick them up now."

NEWS FLASH! HOT OFF THE WIRE!

Nursing intelligence has infiltrated the physician ranks and discovered that rude and dominant behaviors are in fact just a smoke screen devised to keep nurses from ever realizing that physicians are not really demigods after all, but human beings just like the rest of us! This smoke screen technique was started more than 150 years ago when a male physician realized that with a little smoke, he could keep nurses from ever approaching or questioning him. His techniques spread like wildfire among the physician community because it was so effective in keeping nurses "in their place," while boosting physician egos in a male-dominated society. However, having uncovered this top-secret data in 2005, nurses all over the United States are now reporting in record numbers that just one ounce of courage will immediately dissipate the smoke screen!

Remember: These loud and sometimes pompous behaviors are *learned behaviors*.

And the bottom line is when it comes to professional patient care that delivers positive patient outcomes, negative/disruptive physician behaviors are intolerable. The only way to change a culture that has existed for 150 years is to uphold a new standard by a different response—***your response!***

Chapter 14

Going to Mars: Working with physicians, not against them

There are times when nurses come between their patients and the physician, when we feel like we are in the children's game "monkey in the middle."

Your patient tells you she wants to die. Then she shares that no one is listening—especially the doctor. Fill out the "No Code" sheet with signature and witness. Document the conversation in the progress notes. Find out who is the family representative and speak with him or her in private. Simply share with the family what the patient told you and provide support to the family and facilitate communication with the physician.

Families in crises have a difficult time knowing even what questions to ask. Often, they feel intimidated before the physician even enters the room. In a recent *Reader's Digest* article, a physician who was a patient acknowledged that even though she was a physician, she was surprised by how inferior she herself suddenly felt in the role of patient.

A true story of great communication

When the elderly woman arrived from the skilled nursing facility, she was in a Bair Hugger because her core body temperature was 95.7 degrees. The report said she had end-stage renal failure and had been nonresponsive for more than 24 hours. Five elderly children surrounded their mother, nodding their heads as the physician told the family what he was going to do to save their 93-year-old mother's life. No one in the family asked a single question.

Stat orders were given to give three units of fresh frozen plasma, followed by almost a page of additional stat orders. After the physician left the unit, the nurse overheard the family's disbelief that their mother might actually make it through this crisis—they had assumed she would die.

The nurse was not only stressed by the page of stat orders, but was morally upset, as she would not have executed this plan of care for her own mother. The orders seemed above and beyond what would be expected for a 93-year-old comatose patient. She approached the resident who wrote the orders but he would not listen (he was in a hurry to attend a patient in another unit). What's a nurse to do?

The nurse consulted with her charge nurse. Then both went into the patient's room and asked whether there was a family spokesperson. The three then sat down in a private area, with the charge nurse leading the discussion. She asked about the patient's and the family's wishes. The family representative shared that she was very surprised by the physician's orders but that they did not know what to say to him. She asked the nurses for their opinions. The nurses shared with the family member that if it was their own mother, they, personally, would let her die. The woman said again that they wanted a peaceful death for their mother, but that they didn't know what to say to the doctor.

Doctors can be intimidating to family members, as well. In this case, the family representative and charge nurse did some role-playing, and the nurse helped the family write down a set of specific questions they had about their mother's condition—for example, "What are the chances for survival on the current plan of care?" and "What lab values would tell you that this really was the end to her renal disease?"

The physician was paged to the room. After speaking to the family, he discontinued all stat orders and changed the plan of care to "comfort care." The family was grateful, and the physician then wrote orders that ensured their mother's comfort.

A closer look at nurse-physician relationships

Relationships with physicians have been classified into five categories: negative, neutral, teacher-student, collaborative, and collegial. It helps to know the different types of relationships so you can identify a plan and move toward collegiality, where power is equal and your opinion is valued (Kramer).

Neutral physician relationships

Identifying neutral physicians is easy: They see no need to talk to you whatsoever. Like preprogrammed androids, they come to work, perform their tasks, and leave. If you approach them, they look up at you with a face that says, "What are you doing here?" There is absolutely zero emotional investment. Neutral relationships with physicians are characterized by the total absence of a relationship.

Imagine that a relationship is like a doorway. These physicians have shut the door—and some have never opened it. How do you crack the door and let a little relationship in? How do you nudge neutral or teacher-student relationships into a more collaborative role?

- Focus on your shared humanity—share a near miss or clinical error, or invoke laughter by sharing something funny that happened on the unit.

- See that physician as more than a cog in the wheel of healthcare. Acknowledge the time and energy he or she puts into the job. Why is this physician different? What unique talents does he or she bring to the unit? Verbally acknowledge the physician's specific contribution with a compliment.

- Engage the heart and soul of the profession—share a poignant moment about one of the patients. Stories are powerful connectors.

Tip: Insist that physicians that you work with regularly know your name. Remind them if they forget.

Listen up: Dr. Nelson hadn't spoken to anyone all year. One day he came to the charge nurse to tell her a chart rack was broken. Then a month later, he reported a loose shade bracket. The charge nurse joked about his keen eye for mechanical repairs. With The Joint Commission coming in a week, she then asked if he would inspect the entire unit—and he did. As it turned out, he absolutely loved tinkering with mechanical things. One day, she saw a pen that was also a screwdriver in a gift shop and bought it for him as a thank-you. After that day, he was much more approachable and began stopping to talk once in a while with staff. The door had opened a crack!

Teacher-student relationships

Relationships that focus on knowledge are very common in teaching hospitals. New residents actively seek the experience and knowledge from experienced nurses, and this collegial exchange then becomes the foundation for reciprocal relationships when the residents become attending physicians. Teacher-student relationships are characterized by professionalism because they are built on the foundation of mutual respect.

Nurses usually do not hesitate to contact these physicians, and attending physicians answer professionally. But the focus of these relationships is education, and physicians, in discreet ways, still retain their power—which in the end does not empower nurses. Use the tips listed in the "Neutral relationships" section to move these relationships into the collaborative and collegial categories.

Since nurses and physicians getting to know and respect each other beyond the scope of healthcare will build a stronger relationship, joint educational and social gatherings are highly recommended. Another idea would be to have nursing suggest a change in practice that would improve patient outcomes and then share their process improvement with the physicians. By doing so, nurses demonstrate their expertise and build up the level of trust that is the foundation for collaborative/collegial relationships.

Collaborative nurse-physician relationships

The only difference between collegial and collaborative relationships is power. In collaborative relationships, the physician always has the last word. How do you move physicians from collaborative to collegial relationships? This process takes time because the physician must learn to trust his or her team members. Share your powers of observation and suggest changes to the plan of care based on your clinical assessment.

Here is an example:

 Listen up: Elizabeth noticed from reviewing the previous day's progress note that the physician was concerned about a possible postoperative ileus. In her assessment at the beginning of the shift, she noticed that the abdomen was firm and the bowel tones extremely faint. She encouraged ambulation and gave the prn Reglan to stimulate the GI tract. By the end of the shift, her patient was asking for food and his abdomen was noticeably softer. But the physician would never know what she did, as physicians rarely read the nursing notes. Elizabeth charted briefly in the progress notes using the SOAP charting format that many physicians use: subjective, objective, assessment, and plan.

Example SOAP chart

NSG: 7/21/06 7:15 am
S—Pt. stomach hurts
O—Unable to eat, vomited breakfast, abdomen slight firm with
    faint bowel tones
A—Probable ileus?
P—Reglan 10 mg given q 6 hrs. x 2; encouraged mobility/OOB
    qid to chair and turned q 1 hr while in bed

                        Elizabeth Nightingale, RN

NSG: 7/21/06 6:20 pm
Good bowel tones; abd. soft; pt. now tolerating clear liquids
w/o nausea
                        Elizabeth Nightingale, RN

With this written communication, you are literally and figuratively on the same page as the physician. When physicians see a nurse's rationale, insight, and interventions, they begin to appreciate and trust the nurse's knowledge and judgment. This trust is the foundation of good physician-nurse relationships and takes time to build. Unfortunately, most physicians do not read the nurses' notes in the chart, and do not have the time to listen to the daily plan of care—so they really don't know your level of involvement. Show them. To move from collaborative to collegial relationships, nurses must demonstrate and document their skill set to build trust and insist on working as a team to implement the plan of care.

Collegial nurse-physician relationships

Recognizing the different categories of physician relationships is like knowing where the goal is on a soccer field. When you are working with a physician and can pinpoint his or her style, you can see how far you need to "move the ball."

Tip: Accompany the physician during rounds.

Not only do collegial relationships exist, but they are ego-boosting for both physicians and nurses. When a nurse's intellect is respected and powers of observation utilized to the fullest, there is a rewarding sense of fulfillment for the nurse in knowing that it's *her or his* opinion that often makes a significant difference in a plan of care. The reason these relationships are so satisfying for both nurses and physicians is that, in the end, human beings all want the same thing in their work environment: to be respected, trusted, and valued for the specific skills and talents that they bring to their job.

Here's an example:

Listen up: Brenda noticed that her patient's pain had intensified over her shift. She spoke to the patient and then began reviewing the flow chart on the pain assessment sheet. She noted that the pain worsened after the Toradol had been stopped. When the physician arrived for evening rounds he said, "How's our patient?" Brenda explained that the pain had worsened. The physician thought they should switch narcotics, but Brenda had another idea. "I noticed that the pain worsened after the Toradol was stopped. Rather than switching pain medications, I'd like to extend the Toradol for another 48 hours. What do you think?" The physician nodded in agreement. "Great idea, Brenda."

Within this environment, physicians and nurses consult with each other, watch over each other and frequently seek each other's advice, to the full benefit of the patient. This is the goal of physician-nurse relationships. Unfortunately, most physicians have been trained to be commanders who believe in perfection, barking orders at their subordinates. Collegial relationships can only occur when a physician is a leader who knows how to utilize and extract all the human talent around him or her to form a cohesive team. This kind of physician leader knows his or her patients are in good hands because he or she has created the optimal situation for patient safety: a team.

Spin a web of successful communication

Think of a collegial relationship as a complex matrix of fine spider web threads between yourself and the physician. This spider web forms the "fabric" of your relationship. Every single time you have a communication experience that is positive for the both of you (clinical or nonclinical), another fine line is spun. Building this metaphorical "web" is the single most important thing you can do for patient safety. Your web (your relationship) then becomes the sticky trap that will catch a multitude of human errors.

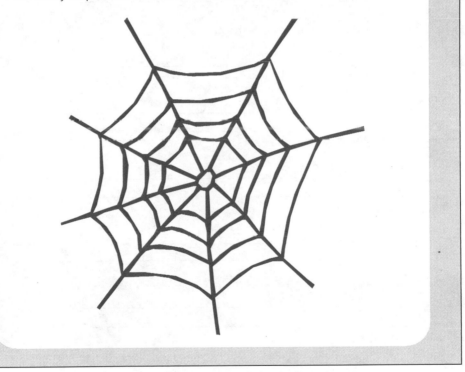

How do you encourage physician-nurse relationships in this category? Being a consistent, honest, and professional communicator sets the stage for collegial relationships. Remember that positive feedback in healthcare for both nurses and physicians is rare. Always take the time to personally thank—or send a thank-you note—to these collegial physicians. Small gestures go a long way in nurturing collegial relationships.

Pulse-taking exercise

In the blanks below, write the names of the five doctors with whom you interact most frequently or who raise the hairs on your neck:

1. _____
2. _____
3. _____
4. _____
5. _____

Now list the above names in the appropriate box:

Collegial

Collaborative

Teacher-student

Neutral

Negative

Pulse-taking exercise (cont.)

And remember . . .
Collegial: Equal-power relationships
Collaborative: Good working relationship, but the doctor has more power
Teacher-student: Centers around communication of knowledge
Neutral: Near absence of any relationship
Negative: Interactions leave you feeling worthless; negative patient outcomes

Possible follow-up actions to above
After reviewing what you've written in the boxes above, make an action plan for improving those relationships. Start by implementing some of the following suggestions:

If collegial, send an e-mail or thank-you note saying how much you enjoy your working relationship. Nominate the physician for an award.

If collaborative, provide opportunities for brief unit inservices to discuss particular cases and increase knowledge base. Advocate for joint education. Attend rounds daily. Perform a review of a difficult case and invite physicians and nurses to it. Form multidisciplinary teams to create standards. Also, send thank-you notes and plan social events to increase opportunities for communication.

If teacher-student, encourage physician-nurse inservices. Include your recommendation for treatment in the conversations. State that you would like to have a more collaborative relationship and that you believe this will help all involved—the patient, the nurse, and the physician. To develop trust and respect, round with the physician and see how your assessment and plan of care compare to that of the physician. Create opportunities for collaboration and socialization.

Pulse-taking exercise (cont.)

If neutral, you must first establish a relationship. Do so by using humor, social events, or conversation to bring the physician out of his or her shell. Encourage conversation and find a common connection. Ask the manager to intervene and have a one-on-one dialogue with the physician. Publicly state shared vision of collaboration at physician meetings. Turn neutral interactions into collaborative interactions.

If negative, take a firm stance on disruptive physician behavior by insisting on a zero-tolerance policy. Hospital or clinic administrators must state behavioral expectations clearly. Create solidarity on the unit. Nursing management, administrators, and physician champions must form a strong alliance. Always try to resolve the situation yourself first. If you are unable to resolve issues on the unit, "write up" unacceptable behavior and copy to peer review. Speak your truth.

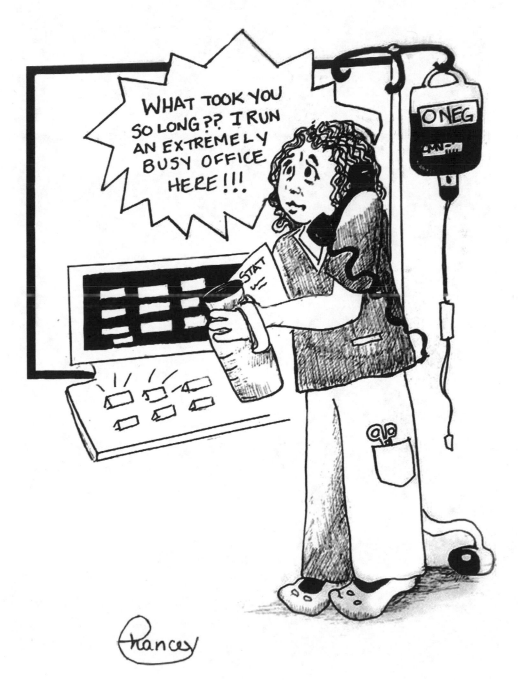

Chapter 15

Dealing with negative docs

Alarm: "The doctor threw the charts down and they fell apart. I asked him to stop throwing the charts and he told me to 'get lost.' I told him that behavior was unacceptable—and he just stomped off . . ."

When communicating with physicians who are negative or intimidating, remember the movie scene when Dorothy meets the Wizard of Oz. Dorothy shivers in fear as the Wizard's voice booms in stereo sound and lights flash dramatically from every direction. Suddenly, Dorothy's dog, Toto, runs over to the curtain and pulls it to one side, exposing the wizard as an imposter. Why, the big, booming wizard is just a man!

Never tolerate any behavior that leaves you feeling like Dorothy did at first—small, insignificant, frightened, or intimidated. How can you "pull the curtain back" on these behaviors? Simply say, "May I speak to you in private for a moment?" Then, state clearly that the behavior is not acceptable.

Listen up: A physician walked up angrily to the nurses' station shaking his finger at the nurse, practically yelling, "How many times do I have to tell you . . ." Instantly the nurse stood up (pulled the curtain back) and said, "Can I speak to you alone for just a moment?"

No physician will refuse this request. It is an expectation, a professional courtesy taught in medical schools.

When alone with the doctor in the privacy of the soiled utility closet, the nurse began, "First of all, I am very bright. And if you tell me something once, I will remember it. I have no idea what you are raising your voice about. And second, don't ever shake your finger in my face like I am some kind of a child. I will not allow this disrespectful behavior to continue."

The physician? He apologized immediately. This nurse not only had a very clear idea of her "bottom line," but she communicated this immediately to the physician. Remember, this story represents a very small group of physicians. And speaking up for yourself gets easier every time. Don't let one bad experience silence your voice and take away your personal power and self-esteem for an entire nursing career.

Tips for communicating with negative docs

If you find yourself in a situation similar to the one in the story above, try these tips:

- Exhibit courage.

- Make unwavering eye contact.

- Possess self-knowledge and self-respect. Know your boundary line, and don't take it when someone crosses it. Period.

- Ask to see the doctor in private for just a moment. If emotions are really strong, disengage until the next day.

- Use the DESC model you learned earlier:

    - **D**escribe the behavior

    - **E**xplain its effect

    - **S**tate the desired outcome

    - **C**onsequences

 Listen up: "In the beginning of my career, I found it really difficult to speak to the doctors. I found out that I must be confident and competent in order to speak effectively with them."

A collection of communication case studies

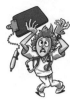

Don't panic: A physician enters the unit and is clearly annoyed and in a hurry—you can tell by her tone of voice and her mannerisms. You need to discuss a concern you have about one of her patients, but she does not acknowledge your presence, and so you hesitate to "bother" her.

The physician will perceive your vulnerability. Don't hesitate or let her behavior change your approach. Be professional and direct. Role model the collegial relationship you expect to have with the physician. Don't hesitate! If you need to speak to the physician urgently, do so immediately by stating your clinical assessment of the situation. If it is a nonurgent matter, wait until she rounds on that particular patient.

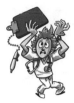

Don't panic: The physician has given you a verbal order—but you do not understand his reasoning.

Ask for clarification. What you are asking for is reasonable: knowledge. There is a six-to-eight year difference in your educational levels. Our nursing practice requires that we know and understand the reasoning behind the plan of care. "Doctor, can you share with me your rationale for this order? I'd like to apply it in the future as well."

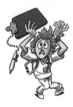

Don't panic: What if the doctor says, "Just follow my orders. You don't need to know"?

You have several options. The first is to say, "I disagree" and then wait for the answer. You could say, "Today's patient safety practices mandate that every member of the team understand the plan of care," or "If I don't understand it, I am not doing it. I am legally liable," or "My goal is to give the best nursing care possible, and I can't do that without using my mind. Or you could use the chain of command: "If you like, I can get you the charge nurse." Tone of voice is everything here—remember your intent and disengage from the power struggle.

Don't panic: There were no bowel sounds at all and the abdomen was very rigid. The postop patient was complaining of severe pain for the third time that morning. The abdomen was bloated and firm. Katie paged the hospitalist who said, "I am just too busy to come see this patient right now."

The nurse said, "Then I need an order for a stat KUB of the abdomen."

"Fine," said the doctor, who then added, "and write in the order to have them page me with the results."

In exactly 40 minutes, this patient was in emergency surgery for a perforated bowel. Her condition was extremely serious. She returned to the floor with a colostomy. If it wasn't for Katie's advocacy, she would not have lived.

Know what you want before you call. Discuss it with another nurse or the charge nurse. Trust your instincts at all times.

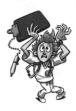

Don't panic: It was 2 a.m., and Cary's patient was still rating her pain an 8 out of 10. Last time Cary called this particular doctor in the middle of the night, he was belittling and critical. After he hung up the phone, she felt awful for the rest of the shift. And now Cary had to call him again.

Never begin any conversation by saying, "I'm sorry to bother you"—not even in the middle of the night. Be professional. You are relaying critical information to the physician on call. By beginning with an apology, you send the message right from the start that you are inferior.

When Cary called the physician at 2 a.m., his tone of voice was once again degrading. She decided to wait until he rounded in the morning to say something. When she saw the physician come onto the floor she asked to speak to him for a minute and said, "I didn't appreciate your degrading tone of voice when I called you last night. I didn't call you for a Tylenol, but for some much-needed pain medication for our patient who was suffering. Please do not speak to me like that again."

Don't panic: "But what if I can't resolve the issue? What if I have tried and the disruptive behavior continues?"

- Speak to your manager

- Fill out an incident report

- Give the chief medical director a copy of the incident report

Don't panic: "What if the doctor is yelling and really hostile?"

Disengage immediately—no amount of communication skill can overcome angry, intense emotions. Walk away from the situation, stating that it is unacceptable. Take note of witnesses. If you need support on following up with this particular physician, ask your manager.

Chapter 16

Speaking SBAR: The language physicians understand

Dr. Michael Leonard, of Kaiser Permanente, and his team examined the different ways doctors and nurses communicated (Leonard, et al.) He noted that physicians wanted clear, concise information and that they were frustrated with nurses "beating around the bush" because in medical school, physicians are consistently taught to focus on the basics ("Just the facts, ma'am").

But nurses are taught to use a narrative style—to paint the big picture. One of the main reasons that nurses use so much "paint" (words) is because they have been reprimanded in the past and told, "You are not a doctor" or "You didn't go to med school, and you can't make a diagnosis." So communication turns out to be a game—with the nurse saying everything he or she possibly can (without ever mentioning the probable diagnosis). Nurses clearly do not feel free to express their needs and opinions to physicians (Leonard, et al.)

This rift creates big problems in communication. "In cases resulting in medical accidents or patient injury, physicians are often noted as saying, 'If she had only told me this was a real emergency, I would have come right in, but I didn't know things were that bad'" (Knox and Simpson).

Alarm: Pam paged the manager. "I've called the doctor three times in two hours asking him to come and see the patient, but he keeps telling me it's just an anxiety attack like her last hospitalization. She is complaining of chest pain, her respirations are shallow and rapid, and her Sat is now 80. He's not listening to me."

Five minutes after the third call, the patient stopped breathing and a code was called.

In an effort to standardize nurse-physician communication, Dr. Leonard and his team invented the SBAR communication tool. This tool gives both physicians and nurses a structure of communicating that meets both of their needs—and therefore, the patients'.

What is SBAR?

Situation (S)	State your name and briefly describe the patient-related issue you are concerned about
Background (B)	Describe the clinical background or context
Assessment (A)	State what you think the problem is
Recommendation (R)	State what you would like to do to correct it

Here is an example of SBAR in action:

S—Situation:	Who is the patient and what is the situation? *"I am calling about Mr. Wright, who is having trouble breathing."*
B—Background:	What is the clinical background and context? *"He is a 54-year-old man with a history of chronic lung disease whose condition worsened after hip surgery. In the past four hours, he has become acutely worse."*
A—Assessment:	What are the clinical signs and symptoms? *"I don't hear any breath sounds in his right chest. His respirations are labored at 32. I think he may have a pneumothorax."*
R—Recommendation:	What would you do to correct the problem? *"I need you to see him right now. I think he needs a chest tube."*

What if I really don't know what is going on? What if I'm just worried?

Say so. If you believe your patient's well-being is in jeopardy, then you must always act immediately. Use all of your resources: the charge nurse, the hospital supervisor, and the rapid response team.

If you are using the SBAR model and do not have a recommendation, seek the advice of the charge nurse or another experienced nurse. It is also perfectly acceptable to say, "I'm not sure what to do. Please come in and assess the patient."

Studies show that a gut feeling usually happens because, at some time in the past, a similar sequence of events unfolded and ended in a bad outcome. So even though just a few clinical events may have happened, your subconscious mind is much more attuned than you think. Trust your instincts.

What if I disagree with the physician? What if I believe the physician's plan is wrong?

1. Reassess and recommunicate. Ask another nurse for his or her opinion. Make sure you clearly state your rationale to the physician.

2. Check in with the charge nurse and ask for his or her opinion. If the charge nurse also disagrees, perhaps he or she can call the physician back and be an advocate. Listen to how he or she handles this conversation.

3. There is always a chain of command. The person above the doctor is the chief of that area, then the medical director for the hospital. And if this is an end-of-life issue, the ethics committee can be very supportive.

Telephone tips

Remember these tips when telephoning a physician:

- Always have the chart, recent labs, and vital signs in your hand when calling a physician.

- Recognize that you may be more familiar with the patient than the physician on call. Be prepared to state all pertinent facts, including how long the patient has been hospitalized, the rationale for surgery or procedures, and *the last progress note by the attending MD.*

- Review what's going on with your patients early in the evening and try to anticipate late-night orders. For example, if the patient's blood pressure has been dropping, sometimes as low as 80/40, ask for PRN orders *before* 10 p.m.

- *Never* begin a conversation with an apology!

- *Always* repeat back the physician's order.

- Remember: *Gut instincts are good enough.*

So what do you want me to do? When the doc wants you to be the doc

Alarm: "Doctors, at times, want me to diagnose and give my perception of the patient so they don't have to come in and can instead diagnose and prescribe over the phone. Other times, they want to manage the patient totally and ignore my perception of the patient. So, I get mixed signals . . ."

Don't get schizophrenic. There are some doctors whose gift of trust and empowerment is decided entirely on the time of day. If it's the middle of the night, do whatever you want. And if it's the middle of the day, don't even think of making a suggestion. If you have this experience repeatedly, write down the incidents and then ask to speak to the physician in private and share your experiences. Don't tolerate the Jekyll and Hyde behavior.

Before an experienced nurse makes a phone call to a physician, he or she usually has an idea of the order that he or she expects to receive. As a new nurse, you are not expected to know everything. Review your recommendation with a senior nurse by saying, "I have a situation that I would like to run by you for your advice." Asking for this type of mentorship builds confidence and skill. In addition, you are following SBAR recommendations, which encourage nurses to think critically and share their thoughts.

But there will be times you hear, "So what do you want me to do?" from a physician. This tone of voice is typically a sarcastic challenge.

Tip: *Ignore* the tone and be professional. Don't let a physician bully or intimidate you. If you know what the patient needs, say it. If you want the doctor to come in to see the patient, say so directly. If you only know the clinical signs and symptoms that alarm you—such as a rising blood pressure—state the facts, and then ask specifically at what point you should call again.

Listen up: "The patient's blood pressure is 190/70."

"So what do you want me to do?"

"I need an order and parameters under which you want to be called again."

After the order is given, repeat the order and ask again for parameters before hanging up. Document the phone call in the progress notes.

Tip: A manager followed up on a complaint that the physician did not return any of his pages for almost three hours. Patient care was compromised. While the nurse filled out an incident report about the delayed return call, she failed to document her attempts to call the physician in the chart. Document every attempt in the progress notes.

Part Four

It's an intimidating word: boss. But it doesn't have to be. This section will help you understand what makes managers tick. It will show you how to work with the difficult ones, how to have difficult conversations, and how to make your working life easier.

Chapter 17

"If I only had
the nerve . . ."

> "It takes courage to start a conversation. But if we
> don't start talking to one another, nothing will change.
> Conversation is the way we discover how to transform
> our world, together."
>
> —Margaret Wheatley

If you hesitate to approach your manager, ask yourself why. *What is the fear or hesitation about? Did you have a bad past experience? Or is it just lack of experience?* Understanding and acknowledging how you feel will set the tone for communication (which is the relationship). Feeling secure when speaking to your manager is all about your level of self-awareness. The confidence that arises when you take care of your own needs will keep you plugged into your own power—which gives you the motivation to form great relationships that will keep you coming back for more.

 Tip: Stating what you want or need reflects a healthy sense of self-esteem.

Managers: In their shoes

> "Never judge another until you have walked three miles in their moccasins."
>
> —Indian proverb

Nurse managers typically do not receive the training necessary to support them in their new roles—especially leadership and business skills. In a system that does not work, nurse managers now need to be exceptionally business savvy—an MBA would be a nice start. They receive constant pressure from both above and below. Admini-stration demands that managers increase productivity and efficiency on their units, while staff begs for more help. Hours of care are in jeopardy every year as hospitals struggle to meet their bottom line, which leaves a nurse manager whose dedicated to both the hospital and the staff in a tough spot. The pressure of trying to satisfy both staff and administration takes its toll.

And then there are some nurses who have been managers for decades but have emotionally disengaged to survive. Staff perceives these nurses' aloofness as not caring, but it is usually quite the opposite. The caring has been wrought out of them. In order to survive, they have gone on autopilot. It is no wonder that there is more turnover in management than in staff nursing.

Whether they are inexperienced or seasoned veterans, nurse managers have one thing in common: They only see the sun on weekends. It's dark when they come to work and dark when they leave. Twelve-hour days every day are the norm. Meal time be-came extinct over five years ago. So did daily planners. Whatever nurse managers intend to do gets shoved aside because of some more urgent issue. Every day begins with a list of 50 things to do. And a good day is when they can cross off just one thing on their "to-do" list.

Complaints from staff, physicians, and patients always find their way to the manager's door. A patient is angry because no one answered his call light; a physician is upset about patient care; and an employee needs time off to care for a sick family member. And after a hard day at work, the manager is well aware that he or she could be called in to cover at any time if staffing is short. During a nursing shortage, there are days when, given a genie in a bottle, the first wish without hesitation would be staffing for night shift.

Being a nurse manager is a lonely job because these employees are separated from their peers by floors, so the only time that managers really get to see their peers is during the endless meetings. The energy that usually sustains group members is dissipated throughout the hospital.

Our chiefs are hurting.

Tricks of the communication trade

- **Think of all conversations as wavelengths.** Your goal is for your manager to understand what you are saying, and then hopefully do something about it (or empower you to resolve the issue). You want your manager to "be on the same wavelength," as you because if he or she is, you will both see the situation from the same point of view. Your responsibility is to try and get *on your manager's* wavelength. Empathy is crucial.

- **Begin by putting out a good signal.** Speak your unfettered truth. The most steadfast and strong signal is the one that comes from knowing who you are and what you want. In your truth, you will discover that your own personal power will come across loud and clear, regardless of the words you choose.

- **Focus on the process, not the outcome.** Your primary responsibility is to tell your story (not to convince, persuade, judge, etc.). Use the DESC model to structure your thoughts: Describing the problem, Explaining the impact, Stating what you want/need, and the Consequence if things don't change.

- **Remember, managers are people, too.** You are talking to another human being who presumably is trying to do his or her best in a challenging situation. If every employee would be willing to create and sustain a good relationship with his or her manager, the unit would be an incredible place to work. When staff members make comments to each other rather than their manager (about complaints, concerns, etc.), there is a general feeling of "nothing can be done about this," which fosters a profound feeling of negativity and helplessness in the workplace. Negativity is virulent.

- **Bring forth important issues.** Managers simply cannot be on the unit 24 hours a day, so they *count on you* to relay important information. They feel valuable if they are effective. To be effective in creating a great work environment, managers must address the issues you are bringing forth. But they can't fix a problem if they don't know it exists. They depend on you to bring concerns and problems to their attention.

 Tip: Your willingness to engage and be genuine with your manager will predict whether the two of you have a superficial or meaningful relationship.

- **Refuse to listen to gossip about a manager.** Gossip undermines intentions and creates an atmosphere of doubt and distrust. Form your own opinion. Create your own relationship. A leader without support is like a ship without water. Perhaps the relationship that you forge with the manager will set a new standard for others to use to communicate.

Chapter 18

Easy solutions for difficult managers

Speaking your truth has been a common theme throughout this book. It is the cornerstone of all communication, regardless of whether the conversation is between you and a peer, a physician, or your manager. You can't make someone care, or force them to give you a schedule that you like. But you can share the effect their behavior has on you and the consequences of their behavior or actions.

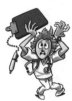

Don't panic: "I've applied to work with my friend at her hospital, but recently she's been making comments about her manager and I'm second-guessing my application. Just how important is my relationship with the manager?"

Critical! It is a well-researched fact that nurses do not leave hospitals—*they leave their managers*. The manager sets the tone for the entire unit. By his or her response—or lack of response—to problems, your manager establishes the standards of behavior for the floor. The nursing leader is the major contributor to morale. Although there are many issues out of his or her control, the nursing leader's *reactions to these challenges* either empower staff or create a depressed feeling of helplessness.

We are facing the largest nursing shortage in history. You have many choices when it comes to where you want to work. If you are not getting the managerial support you deserve and need, you have no excuse but to stick up for yourself—or leave if the issues cannot be resolved. There are plenty of awesome nurse managers out there!

Working for a difficult boss

Interviews are a two-way street. It's not simply a matter of the manager approving of you; it's also an opportunity to see if you feel a connection with the manager and the floor. Is this someone you would like to work for?

The interview process is a perfect opportunity to pick up on some big clues. After your interview, consider the following questions:

- Did the manager exhibit any genuine interest in you as a person, or is he or she just looking to fill a position? Which questions did the manager ask that reflected this?

- Did your conversation with the manager cover your values and vision, and whether they match the values of the institution?

- Did you feel rushed during the interview process?

- What is the manager's span of control? How many units does he or she manage? Does the manager feel supported? (If not, then the manager can't support you.)

- Did you have the opportunity to pose the questions you wanted to ask?

- Did you leave the interview feeling a connection, or was the meeting "strictly business as usual"?

- Did the manager mention the unit's common goal or purpose? (The presence of a clearly stated common goal is evidence of a cohesive team.)

 Tip: The job interview is a great opportunity to learn more about your prospective boss.

Sample interview questions for the manager

Ask some of these questions during an interview to get a better idea about what your interviewer would be like as a boss:

- How many hours do you work in a typical week?
- How many people do you supervise? Do you have staff to help you?
- When was the last time your director asked you what *you* needed?
- What do you like the most about the people who work here?
- What is your greatest challenge?
- May I see your employee satisfaction scores for the past year? Can you share with me your assessment of the results?
- What is your vision for the unit this year? In five years?

What if I'm still not sure after the interview?

- Ask to spend a minimum of four hours shadowing a nurse. Take this opportunity to ask other nurses whether their manager understands their key concerns. What are their major joys and frustrations? Do performance improvement plans exist for the unit? How are problems resolved, and how timely? What is the culture surrounding mistakes? *Every* unit has its own set of challenges in this day and age, but is the attitude generally optimistic?

- Ask to simply sit at the front desk as an observer during a change of shift. You can tell so much just by the way staff meet and greet each other, the manager, and physicians. Is the atmosphere cordial and relaxed? How much human-to-human talk is happening? Does the manager have a good relationship with the physicians?

- Ask to see a copy of staff meeting notes for the past few months. Do the same issues keep coming up again and again? Is any time reserved for staff concerns? Were the minutes easily accessible?

- Ask for the past two years' statistics on employee satisfaction. These statistics benchmark the floor to the organization and to the country. Look specifically at the responses to morale, feeling appreciated, and sense of belonging.

- If the hospital or workplace is unionized, how many Stage 2 grievances have there been in the past year?

- How empowered do staff members feel to solve their own problems? Do they take an active role in finding solutions?

What if I don't like my shift?

Say so. The shift that you signed up for when you accepted the position is your assigned shift. Every shift has its pros and cons. Sometimes nurses think that the grass is always greener on the day shift. But with two meals served, baths, and a new set of doctor orders for every patient, days can get pretty stressful. Evening shifts have less confusion, but also less support—such as pharmacy, managerial, and other auxiliary departments—and you miss dinner with your family. Night shifts have the least amount of interruptions and confusion, and great teamwork is often exhibited as staff members realize they must depend on each other. But being awake all night goes against our natural body rhythm. There are nurses on every one of these shifts who love their hours and wouldn't trade them for the world.

Perhaps you agreed to a night shift, but later find that you are definitely not a night owl. Even after six months, you still find working nights very hard on your system. So, use the DESC model:

D   "I would like to speak with you about my shift."

E   "Even after six months, I am finding the night shift very hard on my body."

S   "I would like to switch to days or evenings as soon as possible. Please let me know if there is a position coming up on our unit."

C   "I feel like I can hold out for another six months, but after that, I will be looking for a day or evening shift on another floor because I really need to respect what my body needs."

Let your manager know *ASAP*. There is a lot of turnover and transition on the units these days. If your manager knows that you need another shift, that knowledge will help him or her when making hiring decisions. For example, your manager may be able to put a traveler temporarily in that position. Here are some other tips:

- Give the shift a fair shot (six months).

- Let your manager know you want another shift as soon as possible.

- Reach out to your peers and be open to relationships.

- Don't go around telling everyone. (Staff may perceive your leaving as rejection.)

- Do let your peers know within two weeks of your departure.

More often than not, when a nurse does not like his or her hours, shift, or unit, the underlying reason is really that the nurse doesn't like the people. You'll find that the greatest job satisfaction comes from the relationships you have with your coworkers and patients *regardless* of the shift. That's why communication is so important—if you can let people know what bothers you, you have a great chance of loving your job. Time and time again, it has been proven that nurses who experience the highest degree of conflict with their peers or managers also experience the highest degree of burnout. So when you say what is on your mind, you immunize yourself against burnout.

What do managers do, anyway?

It's extremely important to understand the role and responsibilities of your manager because it helps you to understand the bigger picture for communication. Middle managers in any institution feel the brunt of the organizational stress because they are pressured from above as well as below. Administration puts pressure on nurse managers to be cost-efficient, constantly monitoring productivity and the unit's budget. *At the same time*, staff members are requesting additional resources for several reasons— patients' lengths of stay have decreased; acuity has increased; technology improvements yield new medications and surgical options; and life spans are increasing.

Above all, the manager is responsible for the quality of care delivered. Other major responsibilities include regulatory compliance; hiring; competencies; retention; and physician, employee, and patient satisfaction. One of a manager's greatest challenges is to hold staff members accountable *while preserving their sense of self-esteem*. Each day brings a new set of unexpected challenges: a code on the floor, an angry physician, a sexual harassment complaint, union grievances, a sentinel event, or staffing for the next shift due to sick calls. Being a nurse manager is a phenomenal challenge.

Yet it was also the most gratifying job I could have ever imagined. The challenge of juggling competing responsibilities is only one facet—creating a great work environment is another. There is nothing more rewarding than the depth of human relationships. Every time nurses have a meaningful conversation, our common humanity reveals itself just a little bit more. Leading staff to truly value and appreciate each other is extremely satisfying. Maybe you too will consider this career path someday!

Chapter 19

Great expectations!

Everybody walks into new situations with a set of expectations that they form from past experiences. But nursing students' exposure to nursing managers is usually extremely minimal during clinical rotations. How do you know if your expectations are too high or too low? Having a realistic set of expectations will set you up to succeed in communicating with your manager.

Professional behaviors: What can I expect?

- **To be treated with respect at all times by your manager and your coworkers.** More specifically, this means that all conversations about your accountability and behavior will be held in private. The tone of voice from your manager is consistently respectful. You are not just a cog in the great wheel of healthcare, but an appreciated member of the healthcare team.

- **A nonjudgmental attitude.** To be given a fair chance to tell your side of the story. Because your manager genuinely believes in you, he or she will want nothing more than to hear and understand every detail of any event from your point of view.

- **To feel supported.** You feel your manager will come to your rescue when you have been falsely accused or when you need help—that he or she will uphold your reputation and defend your actions.

- **To be free to express yourself without retaliation.** You feel that it is psychologically safe to bring up any issue. You look forward to bringing up concerns during staff meetings, knowing that the focus will be on trying to find a workable solution. You feel safe disagreeing with a topic, knowing that your opinion is encouraged and valued.

Professional behaviors: What can I do to help?

- Make every attempt to make an appointment to speak with your manager. The best time is before your shift starts—during the shift is too stressful and after the shift you are often tired and not at your best.

- Always speak up to your manager about things that matter to you. Silence is not golden. It is an old myth that if you speak up, you are a troublemaker. Your speaking up about an issue gives your manager the opportunity to fix it.

- Don't approach the manager on "hearsay" ("he said, she said" gossip). Check out the story yourself first (and the *only* person you can check it out with is the person involved). Validate the problem.

- If you are having a problem with a peer, go to the peer first and try to resolve the issue on your own. Or if you are unsure about how to handle the situation, make an appointment with the manager for coaching.

- When you bring a problem to the manager's attention, **don't forget to bring the solution!** There's nothing a manager appreciates more.

- Communicate routine information by e-mail or in writing (e.g., a scheduling error, equipment issues, and other nonemergent requests). When a manager is on the floor and nurses start bringing up small but important matters, it is extremely difficult to remember them all!

- Try to solve staffing problems yourself first, then use your manager as a resource. If you want a day off, find someone to switch with. Put a note up in the conference room or ask around at report—and remember to return the favor when it's your turn!

- Don't begin conversations with your manager with the words "You need to . . . " Instead, choose the words "I wanted to make sure you were aware of . . . " That is, if you can't figure out a solution to the problem on your own.

- You are expected to contribute to making the unit a better place to work after you have learned your craft. Attend staff meetings, volunteer for a committee, organize a potluck, send a thank-you note to a physician or other departments, etc. Don't count on your manager to be the only advocate for improvement and building a healthy workplace culture. We are all leaders.

Chapter 20

Working with the boss

> *"Our lives begin to end the day we become silent about things that matter."*
>
> —Martin Luther King Jr.

If you have a great boss, then communication flows as naturally as a river runs its course. Conversations happen spontaneously. Your requests are honored, and you are respected as an important member of the team. Your manager is available, easily approachable, responsive, and supportive, and you feel that he or she genuinely cares.

If you have a difficult boss, then trying to communicate is like navigating Class IV white-water rapids while dodging boulders that you never see until the last second. A request for time off is suddenly made to seem like you are asking the entire river to change its course. Problems with coworkers are generally ignored, and you learn quickly that no one is held accountable.

There are as many varieties of experience and personalities in management as there are on the floor with our peers. But the challenge in communicating with your manager is unique because of the obvious power difference: How can I best communicate with someone who has the power to fire me?

And the answer is: **By staying in your own power.**

Stay in your power!

Recognize that it is always more challenging to communicate when there is a power differential. Whether conscious or not, the quest for power travels through the hierarchy of organizations like an alien seeking energy in a sci-fi movie—always hungry for more. When you are in a conversation with your manager and he or she covertly holds authority over your head, the most common mistake is to give away your own power. In doing so, you assume the role of victim. Even if a manager does not exert his or her power, staff members often give the manager power prematurely. All that is required to blast this power-leeching alien into oblivion is awareness—and for some, a bit of courage.

Let's start with one of the most difficult questions to illustrate how to stay in your power. One complaint I hear often is "My manager just doesn't care." Nurses get this impression from past interactions they have had during which the manager's apathy was communicated by choice of words, tone of voice, or aloof body language. Eventually, staff members stop bringing concerns to their manager's attention and "That's Just the Way It Is Around Here" becomes the number-one theme song for the unit.

First of all, not every manager/leader believes that genuine caring is even in his or her job description. Some simply run their units like finely tuned machines where every decision is based on the budget because that's how they were taught or because they are being pressured from above to hold costs down. The male model for leadership is based on authority and data, not the feminine leadership principles of caring and relationships. Today, however, there is a movement to integrate both male and female values into leadership models.

"Where love rules, there is no will to power; and where power predominates, there love is lacking. The one is the shadow of the other."

—Carl Jung

Further, it is a well-known adage that culture is passed down from the top. If a manager does not feel heard, if he or she does not feel cared for or supported, the apathy gets passed along to staff. And from the moment most managers walk in the door, they are engulfed by complaints and problems as if descended upon by a swarm of bees. Nurse managers very, very rarely receive positive feedback from their staff. It is impossible to give CPR to yourself—to revive one's own heart.

Tip: Compliment or thank your manager every now and then—starting now.

That's the big picture—and it helps us to understand more about caring but does not solve *your* problem. What do you do when apathy becomes personal?

But here's what I'm dealing with

Alarm: "When I came onto the unit, Laurie was mad. Her arms were crossed and her face wore a mask of harshness to hide the hurt. 'What's the matter?'" I asked.

"I knew the unit was going to be closed this week, so I tried to help by scheduling myself on another unit. And the manager just chewed me out! I'm leaving. I'm taking a position on the 7th floor . . . She just doesn't care . . ."

How do I confront a manager about not feeling cared for on the unit?

If you should ever find yourself in this situation, the first conversation you must have *is with yourself*:

- Does my manager's lack of caring affect my performance?

- Is this something I can overlook and still be satisfied in my position?

- Can I get the caring I need from my peers, mentor or significant other?

- What *do* I need?

  – Simply to express how I feel

  – Or is it vital that I feel cared for?

YOUR answer to the above questions will determine the course of action:

1. "I can live with this." (However, it was really important that I realized the impact.)

2. "I want to say something." This impacts not only me, but also the morale of the entire unit (Use the DESC model):

    D   "I need to speak with you about the conversation we had yesterday."

    E   "I tried to anticipate the hospital's needs and take initiative to solve a problem. Instead of appreciating what I did, you spoke to me harshly and pulled your weight by saying 'I'm the manager!' I feel like you just don't care."

    S   "I need you to recognize and appreciate the fact that I took the initiative while you were on vacation and that I am a resourceful person who does a great job. I was not trying to do your job—you weren't here (*acknowledging the feeling that would match a comment like 'I'm the manager.'*)"

    C   "I will apply for the open position on neuro rather than allow myself to be treated like a child who misbehaved."

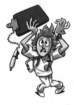

Listen up: Laurie's courage to have a crucial conversation gave both of them an opportunity to heal. The manager shared the additional problems that the prescheduling had caused and why she was so frustrated. Laurie realized her "manager doesn't care" impression was not true. Because of the heart-to-heart meeting, the manager also saw that she needed to show her appreciation of Laurie's autonomy and problem-solving skills. She promised to make her caring more visible. Win-win!

Don't panic: "I can't care for patients all day, every day, without my manager caring for me."

Use the DESC model:

D   "Thank you for meeting with me. I'd like to talk to you about my request for time off on March 25th."

E   "When I asked for time off in writing over two months ago for my sister's wedding, you did not reply. I never heard from you until three weeks before the wedding when you gruffly said, 'You can't have off because we're short.' Clearly, this is an important event, and

I gave you plenty of notice. Your lack of understanding or support feels like you don't care."

S   "I need that date off. Even more, I need to feel that you care enough to help me schedule time off when I really need it."

C   "It's important for me that you understand that this incident has greatly affected me. As a nurse who gives all day long, it is vital to me that I feel supported and cared for as well."

 Tip: When you stay true to yourself, when you say what is really on your mind, you are staying in your own power.

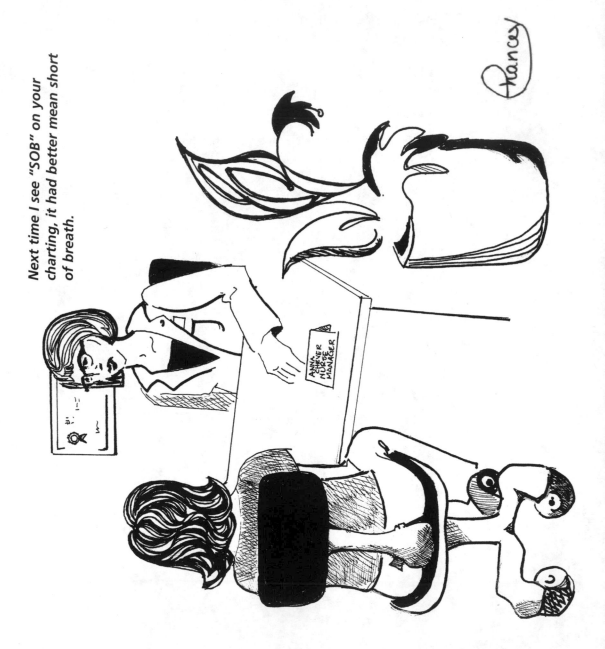

Next time I see "SOB" on your charting, it had better mean short of breath.

Chapter 21

Uh-oh! When the psycho is your boss

Of all the professions on the planet, those of us in nursing have the honor of dealing with the most challenging and interesting people. Homeless, psychotic, frightened, and confused patients are frequently in our care. We provide these patients with generous doses of kindness, support, and understanding. But what happens when the most difficult person in your life is your manager? Commonly seen personality types in healthcare are:

- *The control freak*—"Don't even breathe without my approval." He or she wants to monitor your every move.

- *The authoritarian*—"When I want your opinion, I will give it to you." He or she acts like your mother—when you were two years old.

- *Postcards from the edge*—Definite overload. A nervous breakdown is seen as time off. This type of manager is juggling so many tasks, he or she even dreams of work.

- *The roadrunner*—"Life's a race and then you die." If you can catch him or her, you can have a three-second conversation.

- *Terminal apathy*—Flat affect. No wrinkles. Face is always covered with a blank stare. He or she can't even remember caring.

The bottom line: The better you understand how other people view the world and what motivates them, the better you will be able to influence them to behave in helpful ways (Lubit). This requires empathy—a sincere desire to see the world from another's point of view. Sometimes a manager might be suffering from depression, anxiety, or going through an extremely difficult home situation. Even then, you are not doing your manager any favors by keeping quiet. When under stress, human beings often default to one of the above styles—and managers are human beings.

I, unfortunately, am a roadrunner. When the demands and pressures build up, I just speed up like a movie on fast-forward. My facial expression is intense as I try to concentrate on at least 50 things at once. One day, an employee asked, *"Why are you so mad?"* I had no idea that this was how I was coming across. I appreciate that my staff will venture to comment, because it helps me to realize that I need to slow down. Take five. Stop. Breathe. We all need feedback. Feedback is the mirror that reflects how we are expressing ourselves to the world—if given by someone who genuinely cares.

> *"We can be human only together."*
>
> —Archbishop Tutu

The important thing to remember is that **when these behaviors occur on a consistent basis, it is not normal**. And if you accept these as normal, you will be sucked into the drama as well. "Toxic managers can complicate your work, drain your energy, compromise your sanity, and destroy your career" (Lubit).

There are numerous types of full-time dysfunctional personalities: passive, paranoid, and dictatorial, to name just a few. Care enough to say something and be understanding, but don't make excuses. There is nothing more damaging in the workplace than a toxic manager.

 Tip: Your biggest responsibility is to take care of yourself—your feelings, your boundaries, your needs. Remove yourself from harm's way. Speak your truth.

Tip: For very specific help in dealing with a particular type of difficult manager, check out:

Since Strangling Isn't an Option, by Sandra A. Crowe, M.A.

Coping with Toxic Managers, Subordinates and Other Difficult People, by Roy H. Lubit, MD, PhD

Sometimes it's easier to think of different types of difficult personalities as animals because it helps us not to take the behavior personally. This allows you to concentrate on your response.

Animals in your kingdom

Animal personality	*Strategies that work*
Hostile apes: loud, explosive, and rude; doesn't stop to consider your needs	"Let's discuss our options." Direct and redirect the conversation.
All-knowing owls: can't be right without making you wrong; know everything	"That's a great perspective, I never thought of that. And how about this?"
Sarcastic bees: get a little laugh from the sting	Don't laugh or join in. Get them alone and say "You hurt my feelings." Use great eye contact and be assertive.
Complaining lizards: love to complain; the last thing they want is a solution	Don't nod your head, agree, or sympathize. Say "What would you like to see happen here?"
Unresponsive snails: call as little attention to themselves as possible	Ask open-ended questions. Build a rapport and gain their trust.
The prickly porcupines: classic backstabbers; say one thing and do another, talk behind your back	Either ignore or approach directly. Say "I know you said . . . and I'd rather you tell me directly."

Source: Crowe, S. (1999). Since Strangling Isn't an Option. New York: Perigree Trade. Printed with permission.

Communicating with a difficult manager

Here are some things to remember that will help give you a voice when dealing with difficult managers:

- Remember your self-awareness and self-esteem

- Practice assertiveness skills

- Find and state the common goal

- Don't take the dysfunctional behavior personally

- Have empathy and a genuine interest in a relationship

Self-confidence is a sign of your sense of self-esteem. Confidence comes from knowing your boundaries and your feelings. Knowing that you can hold a conversation with *anyone* and come out feeling a deeper connection to that individual is a very attainable skill—especially in nursing, where there are so many occasions to practice. There is a direct correlation between the extent that you assert yourself and your self esteem.

Tip: Self-esteem is the foundation for assertiveness.

The communication continuum

Passive   **Assertive**   Aggressive

Too hot

Aggression sits at the far end of the communication continuum. Aggressive people try to energetically force another person into their way of thinking. (It's how you shove someone without touching him or her.) People behaving aggressively tend to employ tactics that are disrespectful, manipulative, demeaning, or abusive, and they don't think of the other person's point of view at all. They tend to think the worst of people and quickly jump to conclusions (Scott).

Too cold

At the other end of the scale is passivity, where nothing is worth quarreling about. Every time passive people have a conflict and ignore their true feelings, they betray themselves. Not sticking up for themselves chips away at their sense of self-esteem like a woodpecker, conversation by conversation, until eventually, they can't recognize themselves. Passive people worry more about another person's feelings rather than respecting their own.

Hot and cold

Passive-aggressive people do not like conflict, so they never say anything directly to the person who offends them. Shortly afterward, however, they act out their hurt aggressively by jumping to conclusions (usually the worst one possible) and then lashing out at everyone else. They are afraid to speak up to the person directly involved. Many people who act this way usually had a home situation where they had to tiptoe around the truth.

> *"Assertiveness is the ability to express one's feelings and assert one's rights while respecting the feelings and rights of others."*
>
> —E. Scott

Assertive—just right!

"Assertive people like themselves" (Gaddis). They don't let other people invade their space and are clear about their personal boundaries. By staying true to themselves, they get what they want without the power struggle. **Being assertive simply means you say what you feel.** You do so with respect and the knowledge that everyone has their own unique story. By being assertive, you will have *less* conflict and stress, and *more* rewarding relationships.

Check out this example:

Situation:	Abby comes on shift and picks up her assignment only to find she has four surgeries and everyone else has only two.
Aggressive:	Abby assumes the charge nurse is dumping on her. She goes to find her and says very loudly, "You are so unfair! I am tired of you picking on me!"
Passive:	Abby is hurt. She sits quietly through report and

keeps her thoughts and feelings to herself, knowing the shift will be a disaster.

Passive-aggressive: Abby says nothing. But one hour into the shift, she starts talking to all the other nurses about what a bad charge nurse is allowed to get away with these days.

Assertive: Abby seeks out the charge nurse and asks her if she is aware of the fact that she has four fresh surgeries and the others on the team only have two.

The reality of the situation? The charge nurse never even made the assignment. The day shift charge nurse did and was totally unaware of the huge discrepancy. But Abby would never know that unless she communicated.

Be assertive! B-E assertive!
Here are some more helpful tips:

1. Make sure your body reflects confidence: Stand up straight, look people in the eye, and relax.

2. Use a firm but pleasant tone.

3. Don't assume you know another's motive, especially if you think he or she is negative.

4. Don't forget to listen and question, to understand another's point of view.

5. Try to think win-win: Compromise and find a way to get your needs met.

—E. Scott, MS

> *"Assertiveness is not what you do, it's who you are!"*
>
> —Shakti Gawain

Assertiveness training can be a helpful skill in dealing with difficult managers or other difficult people. Yet one study shows that having great assertiveness skills does not necessarily translate into having better relationships. You may get what you want, but you may still not like or respect the person; you may get what you want, but still feel like something is missing. Keep the ultimate goal in mind. The goal in all communication (whether with physicians, peers, or managers) is that our conversations are the means by which we create healthy, enjoyable, and sustainable relationships. Our words are the bridge to each other.

Want to learn more? Check out "How to Learn Assertive Communication in Five Simple Steps" at *http://stress.about.com/od/relationships/ht/howtoassert.htm.*

A sailing metaphor

Think of a sailboat.

If you have too little wind or not enough sail, you get stuck in a "lull" and the boat doesn't go anywhere.

If you put up too much sheet or have too much wind, you capsize.

For a good sailor, the trick is to position yourself so that you take advantage of the wind you have, putting up just the right amount of sheet and using just the wind to propel you in the direction you want to go.

You want to go—even when the prevailing wind is in the opposite direction.

Chapter 22

Communication CPR: How to resuscitate a conversation

Indeed, when you are dealing with someone who is difficult, additional skills are required. The key is to find the common goal in the conversation as soon as you can because difficult managers often have different or hidden agendas. Think to yourself, "What is our mutual purpose? What is it that we *both* can get out of this conversation?"

This tactic is especially helpful when there is a power difference. For example, your manager might be focused on the budget, so he or she questions the overtime you worked all week. But you *both* want the best quality care possible for the patient *and* for you to get out on time. So redirect the conversation to the interruptions or delays you are experiencing during your shift. Ask your manager to help you identify and deal with those issues so that your overtime decreases.

What gets in the way of this conversation (and all others) are our feelings. Nurses feel defensive, intimidated, etc., because we create our own "story" about why the manager is approaching us before the manager even opens his or her mouth. Be aware of the story you are telling yourself (the reason you think the manager is acting this way; for example, "She doesn't care"). Check out your story during the course of the conversation—don't just assume it's true.

And don't take it personally. Chances are a difficult manager treats everyone the same. These managers keep staff silent by intimidation—this way, the manager never has to deal with the problems of the unit. Nurses conclude that "The manager just doesn't like me," and then avoid all communication. Whatever relationship exists is based on fear. This situation is not healthy for anyone involved. Take the chance and speak up using your new assertiveness skills—or find a great manager who resonates with your value system.

Communicating about hostility on the unit

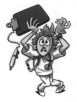

Don't panic: "How do I communicate with the managers about hostility on the unit without sounding like I am complaining or putting other nurses down?"

Hostility is a group symptom. It might seem to you like one person is responsible—and indeed, one person may be doing most of the damage—but the real story is that this particular person has been allowed to get away with hostile behaviors because the group never complained. By their silence over time, the entire group demonstrats their acceptance.

Use the DESC model and make sure you focus on the specific behaviors exhibited and *not* the people involved:

D "I'd like to talk to you about the culture of blame surrounding mistakes on the unit. There seems to be a lot of indirect conversation going on about errors."

E "On several occasions, when a nurse from the previous shift has made a mistake, it is whispered to everyone else on the next shift in hushed tones."

S "I need this to stop. This gossip makes me hypervigilant and sets up other nurses on the unit for scapegoating. It is decreasing my morale and self-esteem."

C "I cannot work in an environment where anything less than perfection is ridiculed, and where the fact that we are human and need to openly discuss errors as learning experiences are ignored."

Dealing with prejudice

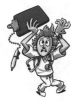

Don't panic: "What do I do when as soon as I walk into the manager's office, I feel like the cards are stacked against me—that she has made up her mind already?"

Sit down and ask if you can start the conversation. Look your manager directly in the eye:

D   "As soon as I walked into your office, I got the feeling that you think I am at fault because your jaw is set and your face looks stern."

E   "This makes me feel defensive and anxious and afraid that the open dialogue I wanted to have with you isn't going to happen."

S   "What I need is for you to listen to me before you make up your mind. I really need your support and understanding. Please, ask me questions."

C   "So that I can tell you what I know and together we can solve this issue."

Combating helplessness

Don't panic: "What about when he or she is 'one of them?' What if you have gone to your manager time and again without results? You've had all the crucial conversations you can hold, and nothing ever changes."

Use the CPR formula to help you move deeper into the conversation:
The first conversation should be about the (C) **content** or the issue.
The next conversation should point to the (P) **process** or **pattern** you see.
If you still have no results, the last conversation should focus on (R) the impact this pattern is having on the **relationship**.

Here's an example:
Let's say there is a lack of supplies.

C   There are no IV pumps. (First time the issue comes up.)

P   "I've come to work every day now this week and have been unable to find a pump to deliver antibiotics." (Second conversation about the pattern.)

R   "I came to you about being unable to find a pump and the lack of the supplies I need to do my job. I need to let you know that this is affecting patient care and leading me to believe this is not a place that I can work in safely."

As in every difficult situation, the person you need to turn to first is you. The key is never to let yourself feel helpless in a situation. There is always power—and you will find it in your response. It's when we don't do something about a situation that bothers us that we sell ourselves short. Ask yourself:

- Why would a reasonable, rational person act this way? Make an assumption and then design a strategy based on that assumption. For example, your manager is very upset. Maybe something happened at home that upset him or her. How would you now approach your upset boss thinking that something must have happened to upset her (Patterson)?

- What would I do right now if I really wanted this (Patterson)?

- What do I want in the long run? Will this action move me closer to that goal (Patterson)?

- Do I think that there is any chance at all that the manager will be responsive if I approach him or her one more time?

- Can I present the issue a different way?

- Do I need to leave my current position?

- Am I willing to go up the chain of command and speak to the director in order to improve the situation?

"*So what is asked of us, the tellers of the new story, is our voice and our courage.*"

—Margaret J. Wheatley

The best units are ones that function under the belief system that everyone is a leader. Your perceptions, feelings, ideas, etc., can help make the unit a better place to work for everyone—but not if you don't or can't communicate what you see and know to others.

More often than not, managers remain unaware of staff members that are angry and upset with them; or of personnel problems and issues on the unit, because no one has the courage and conviction to say something. Find your voice and be that person.

For further reading on the topic, check out:

- *Crucial Conversations: Tools for Talking When Stakes Are High*, by Kerry Patterson, et al.
  (Along with great information, this book contains a test to help you realize your style under stress.)

- *Fierce Conversations: Achieving Success at Work & in Life, One Conversation at a time*, by Susan Scott

Chapter 23

The last straw: Approaching the director

> *"Just the facts, ma'am."*

By this time, you should have had at least three conversations about the same subject with your manager utilizing the CPR communication model (Patterson). Hopefully, your conversations were specific and honest, and clearly stated the influence that the situation was having on your life. Briefly jot down your recollection of the facts. If you want to stay at your current workplace but can't live with a situation, and your manager has not been responsive despite numerous attempts, then your only choice is to go up the chain of command.

For example, let's say there is a recurring problem with trying to decrease the days you work.

C   The first conversation with your manager was about decreasing your FTE.

P   Your second conversation focused on the lack of acknowledgement that this is a crucial need for you and your family.

R   The last conversation you had with your manager focused on the fact that not decreasing your FTE was having a profound effect on both your home and work life, and affecting relationships with both patients and family.

Don't slam, slander, label, or gossip. Just stick to the facts to the best of your ability. Be brief, unemotional, and factual. If your issue is still unresolved after CPR, then approach the director. Use the DESC model:

D   "I have been trying for over a year to decrease my FTE with no success. I have spoken to my manager three times over the course of the year."

E   "My husband has been promoted, and working full time has become a huge stress on our family."

S   "I need to reduce my hours to a 0.8."

C   "And since I have been trying for over a year, I must leave the unit if I cannot decrease my hours. Before resigning, I wanted to see if there was anything you can do to help the situation."

The consequences of not having this conversation (and many similar ones) are severe. The underlying anger and helplessness you would feel from not taking any action will acutely damage your health and your relationships both at work and at home. You are the only person who knows what you feel and what you need. Take care of yourself. Seek out a work environment where you are respected and valued for the incredible gifts and talents you bring to the nursing profession.

Your voice is our future

> *"What we need is what the ancient Israelites called hochma—the science of the heart . . . the capacity to see, to feel, and then to act as if the future depended on you. Believe me, it does."*
>
> —Bill Moyers

"Our natural state is to be together" (Wheatley). There is no award for fierce, "Type A" personality independence, no award for not needing each other. In fact, there is nothing more damaging. And at no time in the history of our profession do nurses need each other more than *right now*.

You are the hope for a profession that currently feels the brunt of a dysfunctional healthcare system but is not consciously aware of the impact. With compassion and selflessness, nurses have spent years focusing their time and energy on their patients. Now, in a global shortage, we must turn to one another.

Take care of each other. Reach out and get to know each other. The pace of our lives both at home and at work has made spending time together much more difficult. Share your hopes and fears, your pride and your accomplishments, and celebrate the art and science of a magnificent profession. It is your relationships that will sustain you and bring you joy, that will bind you into a community of caregivers who care about each other. *This is the most optimal environment in which for you to thrive, and for patients to heal.*

The skills and talents you bring to nursing will carry on one of the noblest professions in the world. If not you, then who?

Welcome to Nursing!

Bibliography

Part 1

"2007 National Patient Safety Goals." The Joint Commission. Available at *http://www.jointcommission.org/PatientSafety/NationalPatientSafetyGoals*. Accessed June 4, 2007.

Anderson, L., and J. Clarke, "De-escalating verbal aggression in primary care settings." *Nurse Practitioner* 21: Oct. 1996: 101–102.

Author interview. Hagedorn, Diane, RN. May 1, 2007.

Author interview. Loughlin, Gail, RN, CHPN, Transitions Clinical Liaison. April 25, 2007.

Author interview. Renno, Robert, RN. May 1, 2007.

Convergent Knowledge Solutions, 2006. Instructor Guide: Communication and Team Skills in Medicine. Weston, Fl.

Dunn, H. (2001). *Hard Choices for Loving People: CPR, Artificial Feeding, Comfort Care and the Patient with a Life-Threatening Illness* (4th edition). Herndon, VA: A & A Publishers, Inc.

Groopman, J. (2007). *How Doctors Think*. Boston: Houghton Mifflin.

Maxfield, D., et al. "Silence Kills: The Seven Crucial Conversations® for Healthcare." Available at *http://www.silencekills.com/pdl/silencekills.pdf*. Accessed June 4, 2007.

Nichols, R. G. and L. Stevens. (1957). *Are You Listening?* New York: McGraw-Hill.

Quinn, J. F. "Holding sacred space: The nurse as healing environment." *Holistic Nursing Practice* 6(4) July 1992: 26-36.

Smith, D. R., et al. (2001) *Controlling Pilot Error*. New York: McGraw-Hill.

Part II

Arnold, E., and K. Boggs. (2002). *Interpersonal Relationships: Communication Skills for Nurses*. Philadelphia: W.B. Saunders

Bartholomew, K. (2006). *Ending Nurse-to-Nurse Hostility: Why Nurses Eat Their Young and Each Other*. Marblehead, MA: HCPro, Inc.

Buresh, B., and S. Gordon. (2000). *From Silence to Voice*. Ithaca, NY: Cornell University Press.

Cox, S. "Good communication: Finding the common ground." *Nursing Management*. Jan. 2007.

Goleman, D. (2006). *Social Intelligence: The new science of human relationships*. New York: Bantam Books.

Griffin, M. "Teaching cognitive rehearsal as a shield for lateral violence: an intervention for newly licensed nurses." *The Journal of Continuing Education in Nursing* 35(6), 2004: 257–263.

Miller, S. (2006). *Conversation: A History of a Declining Art*. New Haven, CT: Yale University Press.

Ramos, M. "Eliminate destructive behaviors through example and evidence." *Nursing Management* 37(9), Sept. 2006: 34–41.

Scott, S. (2004). *Fierce Conversations*. New York: The Berkley Publishing Company.

Part III

Baggs, J.B., et al. "Association between nurse-physician collaboration and patient outcomes in three intensive care units." *Critical Care Medicine* 27(9), Sept., 1999. 206–7.

Bartholomew, K. (2004). *Speak Your Truth: Proven Strategies for Effective Nurse-Physician Communication*. Marblehead, MA: HCPro, Inc.

Knox, E., and K. Simpson. "Teamwork: The fundamental building block of high-reliability organizations and patient safety." Chicago: University of Chicago Safety Group. Workshop handout, 2004.

Kramer, M. and C. Schmalenberg. "Securing 'good' nurse/physician relationships." *Nursing Management* 34(7), July 2003: 34–38.

Leonard, M., E. Graham, and D. Bonacum. "The human factor: The critical importance of effective teamwork and communication in providing safe care." *Quality Safe Healthcare* 13(Supp1), 2004: i85–90.

Rapaille, C. (2006). *The Culture Code*. New York: Broadway Books.

Rosenstein, A. "Nurse-physician relationships: Impact on nurse satisfaction and retention." *American Journal of Nursing* 102(6), June 2002: 26–34.

Part IV

Baldwin, C. (2005). *Storycatcher: Making Sense of Our Lives Through the Power of Practice of Story*. Novata, CA: New World Library.

Crowe, S. (1999). *Since Strangling Isn't an Option*. New York: Perigree Trade.

Gaddis, S. "Positive, assertive 'pushback' for nurses." *The Oklahoma Nurse*, Jan.–Feb. 2007.

Lubit, R. (2004). *Coping with Toxic Managers, Subordinates . . . and Other Difficult People*. Upper Saddle River, NJ: Prentice Hall.

Patterson, K., et al. (2002). *Crucial conversations: Tools for Talking When Stakes are High*. New York: McGraw-Hill

Scott, E. "Reduce Stress With Increased Assertiveness." Accessed April 13, 2007 Available at *http://stress.about.com/od/relationships/p/profileassertiv.htm*

Who said nursing can't be fun?

We're the leading "dot calm" resource
when you're feeling stressed.

 Check us out 24/7 at
www.stressedoutnurses.com

**What will you find there? Along with this
colorful character, you'll see:**

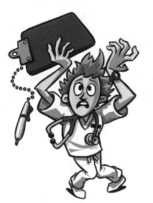

- ✔ **Contests**
- ✔ **Fun, witty articles that will help
relieve your stress**
- ✔ **Resources to help you on your
journey as a nurse**
- ✔ **Much, much more**

So, what are you waiting for?

Get clicking and kiss your stress goodbye!